**Topics on otorhinolaryr**
**head and neck su**

Other titles published by Quay Books:

*Sleep Disorders: a clinical textbook*
by Antonio Ambrogetti, Michael J Hensley, Leslie G Olson

# Topics on otorhinolaryngology, head and neck surgery

*edited by*
*Andrew Swift*

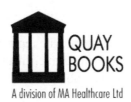

QUAY
BOOKS

A division of MA Healthcare Ltd

Quay Books Division, MA Healthcare Limited, St Jude's Church, Dulwich Road, Herne Hill, London SE24 0PB

British Library Cataloguing-in-Publication Data
A catalogue record is available for this book

© MA Healthcare Limited 2006
ISBN 1856422585

Printed by Gutenburg Press Ltd, Gudja Road, Parxien PLA 19, Malta

# Contents

# List of contributors

Rajiv K Bhalla is Research Registrar, Department of Otolaryngology and Head and Neck Surgery, University Hospital Aintree, Liverpool.

Patrick J Bradley is Consultant Otolaryngologist and Head and Neck Oncologic Surgeon, University Hospital, Queens Medical Centre, Nottingham.

Peter D Bull is Consultant Otolaryngologist, Royal Hallamshire Hospital, Sheffield.

Jim Cook was Consultant Ear, Nose and Throat Surgeon and Neurotologist, Leicester Royal Infirmary, Leicester, and Director, Leicester Balance Centre. He has now sadly passed away.

Alastair Denniston is Senior House Officer, Department of Ophthalmology, Birmingham Heartlands Hospital, Birmingham.

Paul Dodson is Consultant Endocrinologist and Medical Ophthalmologist, Department of Ophthalmology, Birmingham Heartlands Hospital, Birmingham.

Adrian Drake-Lee is Consultant in Otorhinolaryngology, Department of Otorhinolaryngology/ Head and Neck Surgery, Queen Elizabeth Hospital, Edgbaston, Birmingham.

Paul R Eldridge is Consultant Neurosurgeon, The Walton Centre for Neurology and Neurosurgery, Fazakerley, Liverpool.

Giles Elrington is Consultant Neurologist, 119 Harley Street, London.

John Fenton is Senior Lecturer and Consultant, Department of Otolaryngology and Head and Neck Surgery, University Hospital Aintree, Liverpool.

Patrick Foy is Consultant Neurosurgeon, Department of Neurosurgery, The Walton Centre for Neurology and Neurosurgery, Liverpool.

John Hamilton is Consultant Ear, Nose and Throat Surgeon, Department of Otolaryngology, Gloucestershire Royal Hospital, Gloucester.

KJ Harrington is Senior Lecturer and Honorary Consultant in Clinical Oncology, Head and Neck Unit, Royal Marsden Hospital, London.

RGM Hughes is Specialist Registrar in Otorhinolaryngology, Department of Otorhinolaryngology/Head and Neck Surgery, Queen Elizabeth Hospital, Edgbaston, Birmingham.

Nick S Jones is Professor in Otorhinolaryngology, Department of Otorhinolaryngology, University Hospital, Nottingham.

Terry M Jones is Specialist Registrar in Otolaryngology and Honorary Research Fellow, Department of Otolaryngology, University Hospital Aintree, Liverpool.

J Martin is Teacher of the Deaf and Paediatric Coordinator, Yorkshire Cochlear Implant Service, Bradford Royal Infirmary, Bradford.

RL Mendes is Registrar in Clinical Oncology, Head and Neck Unit, Royal Marsden Hospital, London.

CM Nutting is Consultant and Honorary Senior Lecturer, Head and Neck Unit, Royal Marsden Hospital, London

R Palaniappan is Consultant in Audiological Medicine, Royal National Throat, Nose and Ear Hospital, London.

CH Raine is Consultant Ear, Nose and Throat Surgeon and Clinical Director, Bradford Royal Infirmary, Bradford.

Tristan Reuser is Consultant Oculoplastic Surgeon and Ophthalmologist, Department of Ophthalmology, Birmingham Heartlands Hospital, Birmingham.

Nicholas J Roland is Consultant and Honorary Clinical Lecturer, Department of Otolaryngology and Head and Neck Surgery, University Hospital Aintree, Liverpool.

Heike C Romer is Consultant in Pain Management and Anaesthesia, Royal Liverpool and Broadgreen University Hospital, Liverpool.

Andrew C Swift is Consultant in Otolaryngology and Honorary Clinical Lecturer, Department of Otolaryngology and Head and Neck Surgery, University Hospital Aintree, Liverpool.

E David Vaughan is Consultant Maxillofacial Surgeon, Regional Centre for Maxillofacial Surgery, University Hospital Aintree, Liverpool.

# Foreword

Otorhinolaryngology, head and neck surgery is a specialty of great diversity that deals with a vast range of clinical problems in patients from all age groups. Not only do we have such diversity now but there is also increasing pressure for subspecialization, and knowledge will become compartmentalized from one specialist to another.

A selection of current reviews in subjects of topical interest that reflect the diversity of the specialty has therefore been compiled within this book. It is freely acknowledged that the book was never aimed at being fully comprehensive for the specialty. However, topics included are all subjects that the busy otorhinolaryngologist is likely to see during clinical practice, but never finds the time or opportunity to read a concise, up-to-date review on the subject.

Many of the topics that are included reveal the close interaction with colleagues from other specialties that is necessary while dealing with certain clinical problems. Examples include the clinical management of facial pain by neurosurgeons and pain specialists, and the current management plans for both dysthyroid eye disease and migraine. It is anticipated that otolaryngologists will find these articles of great interest, enhancing the advice that they are able to give to patients.

The chapter on how to set up a one-stop balance centre differs from all of the other chapters in that it gives good practical advice on how to set up a new specialist clinical service. The chapter was written by Jim Cook, whom I came to know well as my Senior registrar and who then went on to achieve great things in his Consultant post at the Leicester Royal Infirmary. Jim sadly passed away last year and the chapter stands as a tribute to his good work.

It is hoped that this book will be of interest to all practising clinicians in otorhinolaryngology, head and neck surgery. It should also be of great assistance to those doing their final intercollegiate examinations and other examinations within the specialty.

Andrew Swift
Editor
December 2005

# Chapter 1

# Advances in the management of CSF rhinorrhoea

*Andrew C Swift, Patrick Foy*

Cerebrospinal fluid (CSF) fistulae are underdiagnosed, difficult to locate and often clinically silent. They are potentially lethal and carry a long-term cumulative risk of meningitis. They should be fully investigated and treated aggressively. Current endoscopic techniques combined with intrathecal fluorescein dye enable most defects to be located and sealed with minimal morbidity.

Cerebrospinal fluid (CSF) rhinorrhoea carries the risk of meningitis and is therefore an important symptom to recognize. However, the diagnosis and localization of the CSF leak can be difficult, and there is a significant risk of morbidity and mortality with conventional treatment. Advances in imaging and endoscopic techniques are improving the management and the outcome of CSF rhinorrhoea (Jones and Becker, 2001).

## Physiology of CSF

CSF circulates in the subarachnoid space and forms a protective fluid cushion for the brain and spinal cord. Most CSF is produced by the choroid plexus in the lateral, third and fourth ventricles, and about one-third is formed from ventricular ependyma. The average volume in adults is 150 ml, and the rate of production is relatively constant at 500 ml/day with a pressure of 60–150 mm $H_2O$ (Ow et al, 1999). An increase in the volume of CSF relative to the brain volume is known as hydrocephalus. According to the cause of hydrocephalus, it can be classified into:

⌘ non-obstructive (communicating with the subarachnoid space)
⌘ obstructive (non-communicating).

## Historical aspects

A frontal craniotomy with an extradural or intradural approach is still the standard method of repair of an anterior fossa CSF leak in many neurosurgical centres. This surgical approach, particularly in the acute post-traumatic phase, has a significant morbidity (10.3%) and mortality (2.6%) (Eljamel, 1991). Postoperative problems include:

- ⌘ anosmia
- ⌘ epilepsy
- ⌘ retraction damage to the frontal lobes
- ⌘ infection.

Transfacial approaches for repair of a CSF leak were described in the 1940s, and included an external ethmoidectomy for access to the anterior fossa and a trans-septal approach to the sphenoid sinus. Advances in imaging of the brain and skull base and the development of endoscopic sinus surgery have gradually changed the management of this troublesome problem.

## Classification and aetiology

A breach of the dura may result in a CSF leak. CSF rhinorrhoea can occur from anywhere in the central anterior skull base or from a defect in the middle cranial fossa via the middle ear and Eustachian tube (*Figure 1.1*).

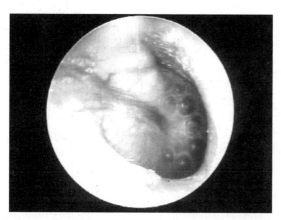

*Figure 1.1: Fluoroscein-stained CSF seen through the right tympanic membrane in a patient with a skull base fracture.*

Approximately 70% of CSF fistulae reported in the literature present with CSF rhinorrhoea, and just less than 30% have CSF otorrhoea (Eljamel, 1991). Eljamel's (1991) review of 253 cases is the largest UK series; it showed that head injury was the most common cause of a CSF fistula (74.3%), followed by surgery of the paranasal sinuses, cranium or pituitary (15.3%) and other non-traumatic conditions (10.4%) (*Table 1.1*).

Within the non-traumatic group, CSF leaks were often classified as 'spontaneous'. However, with improved diagnostic methods the actual cause, such as a small meningocele or a meningoencephalocele, can usually be identified, and truly idiopathic leaks are now rare (Har-El, 1999).

It is important to appreciate that CSF leaks can present many years after a skull fracture.

## Table 1.1: Causes of CSF rhinorrhoea

| Trauma | Skull fracture (affecting middle or anterior cranial fossa) | |
|---|---|---|
| | Penetrating injuries of frontal sinus, ethmoid sinus or orbit | |
| | Surgical trauma | Trans-sphenoidal pituitary surgery |
| | | Skull base surgery or sinus surgery |
| **Non-traumatic** | Meningocele or encephalocele | |
| | Skull base erosion by tumour (e.g. prolactinoma, meningioma) | |
| | Idiopathic dehiscence | |
| | Raised intracranial pressure | |

## What are the risks of CSF rhinorrhoea?

It had previously been assumed that the risk of meningitis would disappear when the CSF leak dried up; therefore, to avoid the morbidity of a craniotomy, the fistula should be allowed time to heal spontaneously. Approximately 70% of leaks cease within 3 weeks; surgery can then be considered for the leaks that persist.

It was not until 1991 that a better understanding of the natural history of CSF leaks and the cumulative risk of meningitis was appreciated (Eljamel, 1991). It was noted that the risk of meningitis continued even when there was no obvious clinical evidence of a CSF leak: the dural defect in such cases had not healed sufficiently to form an effective mechanical barrier to prevent intracranial bacterial infection (*Figure 1.2*).

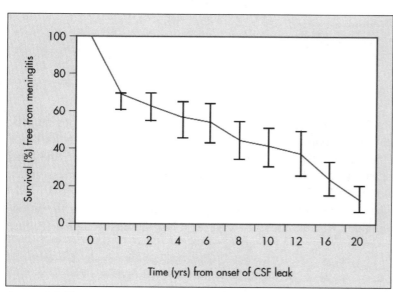

Figure 1.2: The cumulative risk of developing meningitis following a CSF leak. From Eljamel (1991).

This evidence suggests that all patients should be considered for surgical repair, even when the CSF leak appears to have stopped. This goal is becoming attainable with advances in endoscopic sinus surgery, which enables exploration and repair with minimal morbidity. The authors recommend an active policy of detection, exploration and repair of anterior fossa dural defects.

# Detection of CSF leaks

## Clinical findings

The classic history of a CSF leak is a unilateral, intermittent, watery nasal discharge when the head is in a dependant position. Some patients describe the fluid discharge as tasting salty. However, the leak may be minimal or infrequent, making confirmation of the diagnosis difficult. Also, in patients who have had a head injury, the true diagnosis may be a pseudoleak. Such patients will give a history of a watery nasal discharge with exercise or emotion, and the fluid originates from the nasal mucosa as a result of autonomic dysfunction. A watery discharge from the nasal mucosa can also occur after nasal trauma and confuse the true diagnosis.

## Biochemical tests for CSF

Traditionally, the glucose content of a watery nasal discharge has been used to diagnose a CSF leak, but this is far too unreliable to be of any real practical use. The best investigation to confirm a true CSF leak is to test for the protein, beta-2 transferrin (Nandapalan et al, 1996). This test is now available in most large hospitals in the UK. Beta-2 transferrin is detected by electro-immunophoresis and is specific to CSF and perilymph. Occasionally, there is a similar protein in the blood and therefore a parallel control blood sample should be tested at the same time as the nasal fluid. A sample as small as 0.3 ml fluid is sufficient, but even this may be difficult to obtain in patients with subclinical leaks or in patients who are being ventilated in an intensive care unit after head trauma.

## Imaging techniques

Historically, plain radiographs and tomography of the skull base were used to detect bony defects, indicating the site of the fistula. This approach was not accurate or reliable, and radioisotope tracer studies were disappointing. Advances were made with high-resolution coronal and axial computed tomography (CT) scanning aided by intrathecal injection of water-soluble contrast agents, such as metrizamide and iohexol.

Magnetic resonance (MR) scans have also been shown to be helpful in detecting the site of a CSF leak, and T2-weighted images will demonstrate CSF as a high-intensity signal (*Figure 1.3*).

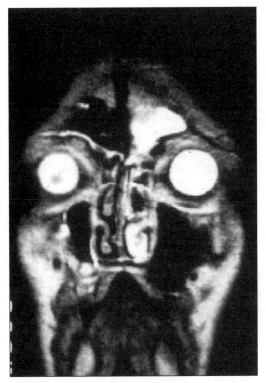

*Figure 1.3: T2-weighted magnetic resonance imaging scan showing CSF leak into the left frontal sinus from an external penetrating injury.*

New generation MR scanners will detect flowing CSF and may well become the investigation of choice. A combination of CT and MR currently gives the best guide as to the site of the leak and any associated pathology, and is the authors' preferred method of imaging (Shetty et al, 1998).

### Intrathecal fluorescein

A small quantity of pure fluorescein injected intrathecally via a lumbar puncture with a narrow gauge needle will stain the CSF a fluorescent yellow. The technique is carried out by withdrawing 10 ml CSF, adding 1 ml 5% fluorescein (or 0.5 ml 10% solution) and slowly re-injecting the fluid intrathecally.

The technique can either be done before simple nasal endoscopy to confirm the diagnosis of an active CSF leak, or before endoscopic exploration of the anterior skull base. Fluorescein takes about 5 days to clear from the CSF, and patients should be warned that during this time their urine will be stained yellow.

Fluorescent, yellow-stained fluid is diagnostic of a CSF leak, and endoscopic exploration will enable the site to be localized (*Figures 1.4 and 1.5*).

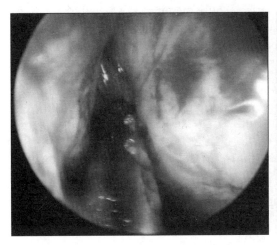

*Figure 1.4: Fluorescein-stained CSF in the right spheno-ethmoidal recess.*

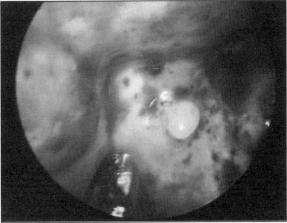

*Figure 1.5: Fluorescein-stained CSF from a leaking meningocele in the right sphenoid sinus.*

Another advantage of intrathecal fluorescein is that it can be seen through a thin dural defect that is not actively leaking at the time of the investigation. A blue light with or without a red filter can enhance the appearance of a minimal leak (*Figure 1.6*).

Confirmation of a subclinical minimal CSF leak may be aided by placing small, labelled, tagged neurosurgical patties in specific sites in the nose for several hours before sending for fluorescein electrophoresis. However, the authors have not found this test to be particularly useful.

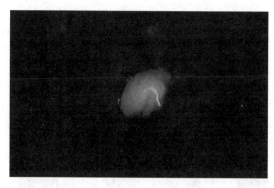

*Figure 1.6: Enhancement of fluorescein-stained CSF by a blue filter in a patient with a small meningocele of the right posterior ethmoid sinus.*

Intrathecal fluorescein is extremely sensitive at detecting even the most minimal of leaks, and although early reports quoted complications, these are extremely rare with modern, purified preparations of fluorescein. None of the complications in the early reports were permanent, but they did include numbness and weakness of the legs, generalized seizures, opisthotonus and cranial nerve deficits (Moseley et al, 1978).

## Management of CSF leaks

### Prophylactic antibiotics

The use of antibiotics in the management of CSF leaks always gives rise to debate. It has been argued that antibiotics do not give any protection against the development of meningitis and that they may actually encourage antibiotic-resistant bacteria to cause meningitis, which then becomes more difficult to treat (Eljamel, 1993). However, a meta-analysis has shown that antibiotics do confer a small advantage in preventing meningitis (Brodie, 1997). It is the authors' view that antibiotics are indicated if there is any history that suggests chronic sinus disease in patients who have CSF leaks from acute head trauma, but they are not recommended for routine use.

### Indications for surgery

Although many CSF leaks will stop spontaneously, there is still a cumulative risk of meningitis of about 10% per year (Eljamel, 1991). Endoscopic surgery will facilitate exploration of the anterior skull base and repair of a leak with minimal morbidity, and the sense of smell is usually preserved if present before surgery (Marshall et al, 2001).

It is the authors' belief that all patients with a recent or active CSF leak should undergo endoscopic exploration after intrathecal fluorescein.

### When to operate

Because of the cumulative risk of meningitis, the ideal time to operate is as soon as possible after the onset of the leak. However, this may not be possible in patients with head trauma until the acute brain injury or other major injuries have had time to recover.

Exploring the ethmoid endoscopically shortly after a skull base fracture will predispose the patient to bleeding and give an unclear view of the skull base because of the inflammatory healing response. The authors therefore prefer to wait 3–4 weeks before undertaking such surgery.

### Techniques of repair

Nearly all CSF leaks from the anterior skull base can be repaired endoscopically after injecting fluorescein intrathecally into the CSF. Once the site of the leak has been confirmed, the surrounding mucosa should be removed and the defect sealed by a graft that is fixed in position by fibrin glue (Tiseel, Immuno AG, Vienna, Austria). Various successful graft tissues have been described and include fat, muscle or fascia from a distant site such as the thigh, or middle or inferior turbinates from the nose. Defects in the sphenoid are best dealt with by obliterating the sinus with fat. Occasionally, a rapid leak that is difficult to control may be managed by inserting a lumbar CSF drain for a few days after surgery.

Extensive skull base defects may be more suitable for external repair by craniotomy.

## Specific or difficult management problems

### CSF leaks after head injuries

In patients with head trauma, the leak may be from either the anterior or middle cranial fossa, the latter presenting via the Eustachian tube. It is therefore important to examine the tympanic membranes with an endoscope to exclude fluorescein staining before exploring the skull base if a leak is suspected (*Figure 1.1*).

If the leak is from the frontal sinus, fluorescein-stained CSF may be seen running as a track from the frontal recess. Alternatively, an endoscope can be passed directly into the frontal sinus via an external frontal trephine. However, the authors have not found this to be as useful as first expected.

A suspected defect in the frontal sinus would require a formal external exploration via an osteoplastic flap. Since this is a much more extensive procedure, surgery is limited to patients with a proven, persistent leak. Whether there is a similar cumulative risk of meningitis from such injuries is not known. However, if a fracture line is undisplaced, it is unlikely that a residual dural defect will remain, and meningitis will therefore be unlikely. Unfortunately, there are no clear answers to this dilemma at present.

### CSF leaks after sinus surgery

With the increased recognition of chronic sinus disease and the subsequent increase in endoscopic sinus surgery, there will inevitably be an increased chance of damaging the skull base. The reported incidence of this complication is low, and estimated to be 0.5% in the UK (Cumberworth et al, 1994).

If a leak is seen at the time of surgery, the defect should be sealed immediately with a graft; nasal mucosa or a section of inferior turbinate is ideal for this. However, if there is extensive sinus disease, a leak may be difficult to recognize. It is possible that such defects may remain unrecognized unless the leak persists or an intracranial complication ensues.

If a leak is suspected in the postoperative period, a high-resolution coronal CT scan should be obtained and, if possible, fluid should be collected for beta-2 transferrin analysis. Endoscopic exploration after intrathecal fluorescein should be considered as soon as possible.

### The spontaneous CSF leak

A small proportion of CSF leaks are spontaneous. However, with the increased visual imaging that is possible with fine nasal endoscopes and the use of fluorescein to detect the true site of a leak, a precise diagnostic cause can be recognized in most cases. Such leaks are usually the result of a small meningocele or encephalocele or, particularly in the elderly, an idiopathic dehiscence in the anterior skull base.

### Recurrent meningitis

A history of recurrent meningitis should lead the clinician to suspect that there is a defect in the skull base until proven otherwise (Schick et al, 1997). It is, however, important to confirm whether the meningitis is bacterial as there are rare instances in which aseptic recurrent meningitis can occur (Mollaret's syndrome).

### Management of leaks from pituitary tumours

Some surgeons routinely repair the defect at the time of trans-sphenoidal pituitary surgery, but others reserve a repair for those patients with a persistent leak.

Patients with large prolactinomas may develop iatrogenic fistulae after being treated with dopamine agonists. Prolactinomas are benign but cause local bone destruction. They respond to bromocriptine. However, as their size decreases, bony defects that are 'plugged' by the tumour open up, leading to a CSF leak into the sphenoid or posterior ethmoid. Transnasal endoscopic repair should therefore be coordinated with their medical management and should only be performed after tumour shrinkage has been achieved (Leong et al, 2000).

## Conclusions

The management of CSF leaks from defects of the anterior skull base has advanced considerably over recent years, and endoscopic techniques of repair are now well established and have the advantage of low risk and morbidity. Injecting fluorescein intrathecally before endoscopy or exploration is an extremely sensitive way of detecting a CSF leak and of tracing the site of the defect. The long-term goal of repairing a defect is to minimize the risk of subsequent meningitis.

## References

Brodie H (1997) Prophylactic antibiotics for post-traumatic cerebrospinal fluid fistulae: a meta-analysis. *Arch Otolaryngol Head Neck Surg* **123**(7): 749–52

Cumberworth VL, Sudderick RM, Mackay IS (1994) Major complications of functional endoscopic sinus surgery. *Clin Otolaryngol* **19**(3): 248–53

Eljamel MS (1991) The role of surgery and beta-2-transferrin in the management of cerebrospinal fluid fistula. MD thesis. University of Liverpool, Liverpool

Eljamel MS (1993) Antibiotic prophylaxis for unrepaired CSF fistulae. *Br J Neurosurg* **7**: 501–6

Har-El G (1999) What is 'spontaneous' cerebrospinal fluid rhinorrhoea? Classification of cerebrospinal fluid leaks. *Ann Otol Rhinol Laryngol* **108**: 323–6

Jones NS, Becker DG (2001) Advances in the management of CSF leaks. *Br Med J* **322**: 122–3

Leong KS, Foy PM, Swift AC, Atkin SI, Hadden DR MacFarlane IA (2000) CSF rhinorrhoea following treatment with dopamine agonists for massive invasive prolactinomas (review). *Clin Endocrinol* **52**(1): 43–9

Marshall AH, Jones NS, Robertson IJ (2001) CSF rhinorrhoea: the place of endoscopic sinus surgery. *Br J Neurosurg* **15**(1): 8–12

Moseley JI, Carton CA, Stern WE (1978) Spectrum of complications in the use of intrathecal fluorescein. *J Neurosurg* **48**: 765–7

Nandapalan V, Watson ID, Swift AC (1996) Beta-2-transferrin and cerebrospinal fluid rhinorrhoea. *Clin Otolaryngol* **21**: 259–64

Ow RA, Syms CA, Gorum M (1999) Cerebrospinal fluid: physiology, drainage and leakage. In: Arriaga MA, Day JD, eds. *Neurosurgical Issues in Otolaryngology*. Lippincott Williams & Wilkins, Philadelphia: 1–10

Shetty P, Shroff MM, Sahani DV, Kirtane MV (1998) Evaluation of high-resolution CT and MR cisternography in the diagnosis of cerebrospinal fluid fistula. *Am J Neuroradiol* **19**: 633–9

Schick B, Draf W, Kahle G, Weber R, Wallenfang T (1997) Occult malformations of the skull base. *Arch Otolaryngol Head Neck Surg* **123**(1): 77–80

# Chapter 2

# Neurosurgery and facial pain

*PR Eldridge*

This article reviews the diagnosis, differential diagnosis and management of trigeminal neuralgia, the commonest facial pain condition treated by the neurosurgeon. The advantages offered by microvascular decompression as a treatment are reviewed and compared with medical treatment and percutaneous techniques.

There are many causes of facial pain, but only trigeminal neuralgia (TGN) is predominantly managed neurosurgically; consequently, most of this article covers this condition. TGN has become famous because of its association with arterial compression at the root entry zone, and the observation that the pain is apparently 'cured' by moving this vessel away. Thus, it is an unusual example of a chronic pain corrected by a surgical procedure designed to remove the cause. TGN is the best understood of a number of neurovascular compression syndromes; of the other conditions only glossopharyngeal neuralgia and possibly geniculate neuralgia present with pain, although the next commonest condition treated is hemifacial spasm.

## Trigeminal neuralgia

### Incidence and prevalence

The incidence of TGN is estimated to be 50/million/year and the prevalence at 155/100 000. Frequency increases with age. Between 2–4% of multiple sclerosis (MS) cases suffer from TGN, while 5% of cases of TGN are in association with MS (Nurmikko and Eldridge, 2001).

### Cause of trigeminal neuralgia

Just after the trigeminal nerve leaves the pons, there is a junctional area between the central and peripheral myelin, measuring about half a centimetre, which is termed the root entry zone (*Figure 2.1*).

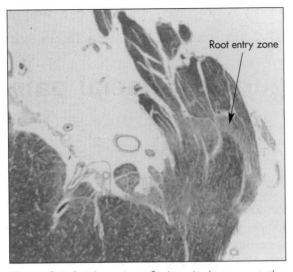

Root entry zone

Figure 2.1: Axial section of trigeminal nerve at the pons showing the root entry zone.

Four observations argue that contact by a vessel at the root entry zone is a major cause of TGN (Miles et al, 1997; Leandri et al, 1998):

- In over 90% of cases a vessel, usually an artery (rarely a vein), is found in contact with or grooving the trigeminal nerve as it exits the pons
- The usual outcome of microvascular decompression (MVD) is instantaneous pain relief
- Intraoperative recordings demonstrate recovery of nerve conduction and far-field evoked potentials
- Sensory function improves following decompression, although this takes up to 6 months.

The mechanism by which vascular compression or contact causes TGN is unclear, including the reason why the root entry zone is sensitive to the effects of vascular contact. Demyelination of the nerve at the position of vascular contact has been reported and linked with the observation that where plaques occur in the trigeminal system, TGN is found in sufferers of MS (Nurmikko and Eldridge, 2001). However, this does not explain the intermittent nature of the condition, its paroxysmal quality and neither the phenomenon of triggering nor that not all individuals with contacts experience pain. Hence, in order to explain these features it is further proposed that in TGN spontaneous discharges occur within a hyperexcitable trigeminal ganglion (Rappaport and Devor, 1994).

### Clinical features

Unilateral, sharp, stabbing or 'electric shock-like' paroxysmal pain is felt in the distribution of one or more branches of the trigeminal nerve. The pain may be triggered by touching the face, chewing, talking or by wind on the face, leading to a tendency for the condition to be worse in winter. The pain is intermittent in nature, with remissions lasting several weeks or months. The response to carbamazepine is so typical that its absence should question the diagnosis, being careful not to confuse lack of response with intolerance of the drug. The pain is refractory to aspirin, paracetamol, non-steroidal anti-inflammatory agents and opioids. In the majority of cases, the pain involves the second or third divisions of the trigeminal nerve, and only relatively rarely is the pain purely in the first division.

## Signs

In classical teaching, there are no signs, although a decreased corneal reflex may occur. Therefore, any neurological deficit found on bedside testing should raise the suspicion of a structural lesion or of idiopathic trigeminal neuropathy. However, quantitative sensory testing carried out under laboratory conditions will reveal sensory deficits (Bowsher et al, 1997).

## Differential diagnosis

Differential diagnosis includes a spectrum of other facial pain and headache syndromes but rarely temporal arteritis or pain radiating from the neck. Patients rarely present with dental pain to the neurosurgical clinic, perhaps surprisingly, although a large number of patients with TGN have first passed through a dental practice. The conditions that cause most difficulty are:

⌘ atypical facial pain
⌘ cluster headache
⌘ painful trigeminal neuropathy
⌘ temporomandibular joint (TMJ) dysfunction
⌘ postherpetic neuralgia
⌘ dysaesthetic facial pain.

### Atypical facial pain

This is a variant of depression, and other features of depression will be present. The pain is continuous, not paroxysmal. The patient is often unshakably convinced of an organic cause. Pain descriptors are often modified to fit one or more of the other syndromes described below; in this Internet age, the patient may be well informed, ascribing great importance to matters of minute detail. This can be an extremely difficult condition to manage.

### Cluster headache

This is regarded as a variant of migraine, and is a vascular headache. Attacks are stereotyped and are clustered in time and space. Autonomic features such as a congested nose or watering eyes may be present. The condition is provoked by alcohol and may be relieved by triptans, which may need intramuscular administration because of the time course of the action of the triptans.

### Painful trigeminal neuropathy

This describes pain from structural lesions, such as the extremely rare trigeminal schwannoma or lesions in the region of the cavernous sinus. Although classically described as TGN, the pain is different, being continuous, progressive and associated with neurological deficit. Idiopathic painful trigeminal neuropathy describes these features when no structural lesion can be identified.

### TMJ dysfunction

This is perhaps better viewed as a myofascial pain involving the temporalis muscle. It is provoked and aggravated, but not triggered, by chewing. True disorders of the TMJ do occur, but are rarer.

### Postherpetic neuralgia

This is rare, usually involves the forehead and follows an attack of herpes. Allodynia is often present in the affected area.

### Dysaesthetic facial pain

This is a neuropathic pain resulting from nerve injury, and is most often seen as a side effect of lesioning techniques for TGN (e.g. as the foramen ovale methods or alcohol peripheral neurectomy). It is a continuous burning pain, which at its worst is termed anaesthesia dolorosa, when it is virtually untreatable.

Differential diagnosis can be difficult and relies most of all on the clinical history. Leading questions by the doctor are a hazard; also, the patient's description of the pain may not be consistent. There is great merit in seeing the patient on more than one occasion to avoid this problem.

### Investigations

No specific test exists for the condition. Magnetic resonance imaging (MRI) detects the presence or absence of neurovascular contact at the root entry zone with a sensitivity of 100% and specificity of 96% validated in a series of 55 cases (Meaney et al, 1995) (*Figure 2.2*).

As neurovascular contact occurs in 10% of controls, MRI cannot be sensitive or specific for the diagnosis of TGN, and the role of MRI is to aid choices for management.

Attempts have been made to demonstrate preoperatively neurophysiological abnormalities, particularly far-field evoked potentials, but these have not proven to be either sufficiently sensitive or specific.

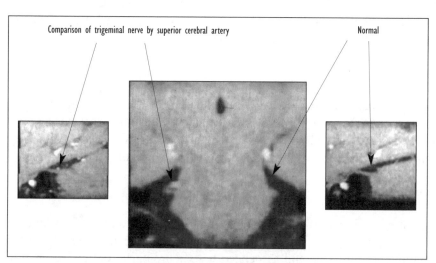

Comparison of trigeminal nerve by superior cerebral artery      Normal

*Figure 2.2: Magnetic resonance imaging showing unilateral arterial compression in the coronal plane and in sagittal reformats along the line of the nerve.*

# Management

## *Natural history*

The natural history of the condition is for the severity of attacks to worsen and for the periods of remission to shorten. Symptomatically, the syndrome may evolve from its typical form to an atypical form in which there is a constant background burning element to the pain, in addition to the classical features (Burchiel and Slavin, 2000; Nurmikko and Eldridge, 2001).

## *Medical management*

The drug of first choice, as mentioned above, is carbamazepine. Although it is effective, this treatment is not without problems. It is difficult to estimate accurately the numbers of patients who 'fail' medical treatment. Reasons for failure are idiosyncratic reactions to carbamazepine (a rash being typical) and dose-related problems. At a high dose (actioned by the severity of the pain) there may be ataxia and severe drowsiness. However, the cognitive impairment produced by the drug is underestimated, and may be the principal reason why some sources have found failure rates with carbamazepine reaching 75% of cases treated. One long-term study over 10 years showed that either loss of effect or intolerance occurred in over 50% of patients (Taylor et al, 1981).

Effective alternatives include lamotrigine, phenytoin, sodium valproate and gabapentin. All these are used in the author's practice and found to be effective in combination, although there is no published study comparing monotherapy and polytherapy.

Some reports, but not in the author's practice, have found baclofen to be effective.

Medication should be withdrawn gradually because of the risk of provoking a seizure (although this rarely occurs). Sodium valproate and phenytoin find application in the acute situation as they can be given intravenously.

## *Foramen ovale methods*

## *Radiofrequency lesioning*

A needle is introduced via the foramen ovale, and electrical stimulation is performed to confirm correct placement of the needle by inducing paraesthesiae in that area of the face in which the TGN is occurring. The patient is then anaesthetized, and a thermocoagulation is performed (60–90 °C for approximately 45 seconds). It was originally suggested that heat preferentially destroyed thin pain fibres, but formal sensory testing finds that all fibres are affected approximately equally. It is difficult to target the ophthalmic division, and this runs the risk of corneal anaesthesia. Masseter weakness is a further risk.

Over 90% of patients experience immediate relief of pain. However, with time there is a gradual recurrence. Recurrence rates vary with series, ranging from as poor as 25% pain free at 2 years, up to 80% pain free (Taha et al, 1995; Yoon et al, 1999), and seem to be related to the technique. If deep hypalgesia is produced during the procedure, essentially by creating a larger lesion, the recurrence rate is lower. Unfortunately, the larger the lesion, the greater the risk of creating dysaesthesias and the feared complication of anaesthesia dolorosa. In series with low recurrence rates, a higher dysaesthesia rate is found; in the worst series as much as 25% of cases will exhibit dysaesthesia, which the patient regards as unpleasant but tolerable. However, in 8% of patients, quality-of-life assessment after treatment indicates that although the original TGN is controlled, overall quality of life is unchanged. In 1% there is severe disabling anaesthesia dolorosa. The procedure is regarded as safe but not completely risk free. It involves intermittent anaesthesia in an elderly patient, and reported complications include meningitis and caroticocavernous fistulae (Taha et al, 1995; Tronnier et al, 2001).

### Glycerol

A needle is again placed into the foramen ovale, and glycerol is introduced under fluoroscopic control. Accurate positioning of the needle is important. The technique has caused much controversy. In the hands of its proponents, excellent results are obtained (best reports being 90% pain free at 1 year). However, others report poor results (only 17% pain free at 5 years at worst) with significant dysaesthesia rates, reaching 44% in some series (Nurmikko and Eldridge, 2001).

### Balloon microcompression

This is performed under general anaesthesia. A Fogarty catheter is passed into Meckel's cave and inflated for between 1–6 minutes. Sensory impairment is produced, although this is mild. The best reported results indicate a recurrence in around one third of cases, with a dysaesthesia rate of around 10%. However, some find a much higher recurrence rate and regard it as a temporary treatment with the advantage of producing almost no dysaesthesia. In a comparative study, 44% of patients were pain free at 2 years following balloon microcompression, while similar figures were 58% for radiofrequency (RF) lesioning and 75% for MVD; it was concluded that the latter is the treatment of choice (Meglio et al, 1990).

### Surgical management

### Operation

This is performed via a retromastoid craniectomy (*Figure 2.3*). The subsequent approach is over the surface of the cerebellum until the nerve is identified (*Figure 2.4*). Arteries must be dissected free and held clear from the nerve using a small piece of Ivalon sponge or Teflon. If a vein is the cause, it may be coagulated and divided. If no vessel is found, a partial sensory rhizotomy gives good relief as being a centrally placed lesion it seems less likely to cause anaesthesia dolorosa.

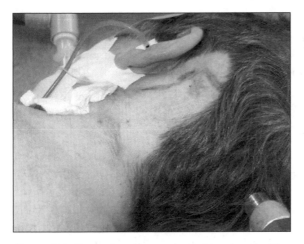

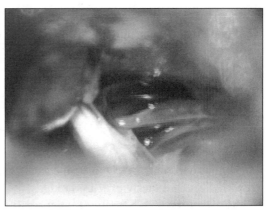

*Figure 2.3: Operative approach and landmarks. The lateral and sigmoid sinus are marked. The star marks the position of the craniectomy.*

*Figure 2.4: Operative view showing trigeminal nerve with superior cerebellar artery lying in typical position medial to nerve in the angle between it and the pons.*

### Risks

In most published series, the serious morbidity (death or major stroke) is significantly below 1% (Barker et al, 1996). As the operation is performed near the acoustic nerve, it also carries a risk of hearing impairment, possibly as a result of traction on the nerve while retracting structures to gain access to the deeper trigeminal nerve. Since brainstem auditory-evoked responses have been used as a monitoring device peroperatively, the risk of unintentional hearing deficit has been reduced to about 2–3% from historical series, where risks might be as high as 13%.

### Outcomes

Overall, excellent long-term results are obtained in about 90% of patients with clear arterial compression, of whom some 70% are completely pain free and off medication up to 20 years postoperatively. Results of venous compression are less good, as are the outcomes following partial rhizotomy (approximately 60–70% at 2-year follow-up). Case selection is important, as poor outcomes from MVD are found in patients with atypical pain or in whom the diagnosis is not TGN. Prior RF lesioning may leave the patient with dysaesthesia, revealed by successful MVD (Hunn et al, 1998).

### Stereotactic radiosurgery

Some controversy surrounds the results of stereotactic radiosurgery, where focused radiation is applied to the root entry zone using the gamma knife, although there is no reason why a suitably equipped linear accelerator stereotactic system should not be used. Unfortunately, the tendency of units is to report results as 'good' and not to specify the true 'pain-free and off medication' outcome rate used in other techniques. When this stricter criterion is used, results are less impressive: only 65% of patients experience pain relief at 6 months, rising to 75% at 33 months. Thus the effect is not immediate. Furthermore, only 56% of those achieving relief continued to have complete or partial relief at 5 years' follow-up, implying a high recurrence rate. There is a dysaesthesia rate and also a dose-related post-radiation numbness (Maesawa et al, 2001).

## Choice of technique

The author considers MVD to be the treatment of choice in most instances of severe TGN, while recognizing that other views are held.

MVD corrects a structural abnormality and is the only technique that effects a cure. Neurophysiologically, the patient is returned to normal, whereas other methods depart from normal, being destructive lesions. The risk of all destructive lesions is neuropathic pain, at its worst anaesthesia dolorosa. The habit of performing peripheral nerve avulsions or alcohol injections is associated with an almost universal recurrence and a high incidence of late dysaesthetic pains.

The following points support the use of MVD:

⌘ The natural history is for the condition to worsen
⌘ Medical management has significant side effects, and most patients fail this treatment
⌘ MVD is demonstrated to be effective and of low risk, including in the elderly population
⌘ In no series does the efficacy of RF lesioning surpass that of MVD, and in the case of radio-surgery the efficacy is poorer
⌘ Results from MVD are poorer after failed percutaneous procedures
⌘ All destructive lesions (peripheral, foramen ovale, radiosurgery) are associated with a significant recurrence rate, incidence of sensory deficit and production of unpleasant dysaesthetic symptoms or even anaesthesia dolorosa
⌘ The sensitivity and specificity of MRI to detect neurovascular compression is such that patients with arterial compression can be advised of the likelihood of an excellent outcome, and patients can be offered an alternative technique if the scan is negative
⌘ Although no randomized controlled studies exist, the authors of two comparative studies concluded that MVD is the treatment of choice (Meglio et al, 1990; Tronnier et al, 2001).

## Fitness for surgery

Because MVD involves craniectomy and TGN occurs in elderly people, fitness for surgery is an issue. However, series exist in which there is little difference in outcome or morbidity when comparing an over 70-year-old age group with a younger age group (Javadpour et al, 2000). Few patients are unsuitable for this procedure with modern anaesthesia, and the choice between percutaneous RF lesioning and MVD can be based solely on the outcomes of the procedures. It is worth remembering that RF lesioning and balloon microcompression both require general anaesthesia.

If a foramen ovale method is to be used, the author considers that the choice between balloon, radiofrequency and glycerol is best made according to that technique with which the treating physician is most experienced; however, the author currently prefers balloon microcompression.

### Trigeminal neuralgia as an emergency

Occasionally, patients present as an emergency with severe pain. The patient is drowsy and ataxic, having by this point taken so much carbamazepine as to suffer severe toxic effects, and is furthermore dehydrated, being unable to swallow fluids because this action is triggering the neuralgia.

Management requires admission and bed rest for the ataxia, intravenous fluids to correct dehydration and finally measures to treat the pain. An intravenous loading dose of either phenytoin or sodium valproate is usually effective in treating the pain. This may be followed by emergency MVD or, if MRI is negative for compression, one of the foramen ovale methods.

# Glossopharyngeal neuralgia

In reality, the anatomy of the lower cranial nerves is such that the glossopharyngeal nerve may be considered as the upper part of a complex that includes itself, the vagus and the cranial part of the accessory nerve.

The syndrome may be considered as identical to TGN, except in two aspects: first it is considerably rarer; and second the pain is distributed in the area of the glossopharyngeal nerve. Thus, the shooting pain is more within the throat, and triggering is also from the back of the throat. Treatment is identical, with the firstline drug being carbamazepine, and surgical decompression providing much the same results as for TGN. There is no equivalent to RF lesioning in this condition.

# VII/VIII complex

Hemifacial spasm, tinnitus and nervus intermedius neuralgia arise from this complex. MVD is effective for hemifacial spasm, which is the most common manifestation of compression at this level. The procedure for tinnitus is rarely performed and controversial, while pure nervus intermedius neuralgia is extremely rare. It can present with otalgia or throat pain (Rupa et al, 1991).

# References

Barker FG, Jannetta PJ, Bissonette DJ, Larkins MV, Jho HD (1996) The long-term outcome of microvascular decompression for trigeminal neuralgia. *N Engl J Med* **334**: 1077–83

Bowsher D, Miles JB, Haggett CE, Eldridge PR (1997) Trigeminal neuralgia: a quantitative sensory perception threshold study in patients who had not undergone previous invasive procedures. *J Neurosurg* **86**(2): 190–2

Burchiel KJ, Slavin KV (2000) On the natural history of trigeminal neuralgia. *Neurosurgery* **46**(1): 152–5

Hunn MK, Eldridge PR, Miles JB, West B (1998) Persistent facial pain following microvascular decompression of the trigeminal nerve. *Br J Neurosurg* **12**(1): 23–8

Javadpour M, Eldridge PR, Varma TRK, Weaver A, Nurmikko T, Miles JB (2000) Microvascular decompression for trigeminal neuralgia in patients over the age of 70 years. *Acta Neurochir* **142**: 1182

Leandri M, Eldridge P, Miles J (1998) Recovery of nerve conduction following microvascular decompression for trigeminal neuralgia. *Neurology* **51**(6): 1641–6

Maesawa S, Salame C, Flickinger JC, Pirris S, Kondziolka D, Dunsford LD (2001) Clinical outcomes after stereotactic radiosurgery for idiopathic trigeminal neuralgia. *J Neurosurg* **94**: 14–20

Meaney JF, Eldridge PR, Dunn LT, Nixon TE, Whitehouse GH, Miles JB (1995) Demonstration of neurovascular compression in trigeminal neuralgia with magnetic resonance imaging. *J Neurosurg* **83**: 799–805

Meglio M, Cioni B, Moles A, Visocchi M (1990) Microvascular decompression *vs* percutaneous procedures for typical trigeminal neuralgia: personal experience. *Stereotactic Functional Neurosurgery* **54-55**: 76–9

Miles JB, Eldridge PR, Haggett CE, Bowsher D (1997) Sensory effects of microvascular decompression in trigeminal neuralgia. *J Neurosurg* **86**(2): 193–6

Nurmikko TJ, Eldridge PR (2001) Trigeminal neuralgia: pathophysiology, diagnosis and current treatment. *Br J Anaesth* **87**(1): 117–32

Rappaport ZH, Devor M (1994) Trigeminal neuralgia: the role of self-sustaining discharge in the trigeminal ganglion. *Pain* **56**: 127–38

Rupa V, Saunders RL, Weider DJ (1991) Geniculate neuralgia: the surgical management of primary otalgia. *J Neurosurg* **75**: 505–11

Taha JM, Tew JM, Buncher CR (1995) A prospective 15-year follow up of 154 consecutive patients with trigeminal neuralgia treated by percutaneous stereotactic radiofrequency thermal rhizotomy. *J Neurosurg* **83**: 989–93

Taylor JC, Brauer S, Espir MLE (1981) Long-term treatment of trigeminal neuralgia with carbamazepine. *Postgrad Med J* **57**: 16–18

Tronnier VM, Rasche D, Hamer J, Kienle A-L, Kunze S (2001) Treatment of idiopathic trigeminal neuralgia: comparison of long-term outcome after radiofrequency rhizotomy and microvascular decompression. *Neurosurgery* **48**: 1261–8

Yoon KB, Wiles JR, Miles JB, Nurmikko TJ (1999) Long-term outcome of percutaneous thermocoagulation in trigeminal neuralgia. *Anaesthesia* **54**: 803–8

# Chapter 3

# Classification and diagnosis of facial pain

*Nick S Jones*

This is an interesting time to consider the classification of facial pain because of the emergence of new ideas that challenge our understanding of the mechanisms involved. The new hypotheses that have been proposed appear to be of clinical relevance.

Great efforts have been made to categorize facial pain into diagnostic categories based on either the symptoms, signs or aetiology. This approach has classified patients in an effort to understand the aetiology and thus find the most effective treatment for each group. The last specific consensus document was produced 13 years ago (Headache Classification Committee of the International Headache Society (IHS), 1988), and pointed out that it was difficult to have definitions rather than descriptions. Some diagnoses have relatively tight descriptions, such as trigeminal neuralgia or cluster headache, but even these have no diagnostic tests. The current alternative classifications (*Table 3.1*), although laudable in their aim to help research and treatment, are undermined in practice because many patients cannot be classified into one or more distinct diagnostic groups. Treatment selection is then based on the category the patients resemble closest, and the best treatment for that group.

## Classification of facial pain

Have there been any advances recently? Ideas from the Copenhagen group (Olesen, 1991; Olesen and Rasmussen, 1995; Bendtsen et al, 1996; Jensen, 1999; Bendtsen, 2000; Jensen and Olesen, 2000) on tension-type headache have resulted in a model that may be relevant to other patients with facial pain. While tension-type headache describes a group of symptoms with some broad but inconsistent features, these theories provide a more inclusive, encompassing interpretation of its aetiology. Essentially, these theories expound central sensitization of the trigeminal nucleus from:

⌘ Prolonged nociceptive input from a peripheral injury, surgery or inflammation
⌘ Pericranial myofascial nociceptive input
⌘ Psychological or neurological factors reducing supraspinal inhibition.

**Table 3.1: Comparison of the International Headache Society (Headache Classification Committee of the IHS, 1988) and International Association for the Study of Pain (IASP) (1994) classifications**

| IHS classification | IASP classification |
|---|---|
| 1. Migraine | Group V: primary headache syndromes, vascular disorders and cerebrofluid syndromes |
| 1.1 Migraine without aura | |
| 1.2 Migraine with aura | Migraine, common migraine |
| 1.2.1 Migraine with typical aura | Migraine variants |
| 1.2.2 Migraine with prolonged aura more subgroups) | Mixed headache (more in group V later) |
| 2. Tension-type headache | Group III: craniofacial pain of musculoskeletal origin |
| 2.1 Episodic tension-type headache (more subgroups) | Acute tension headache |
| 2.2 Chronic tension-type headache (more subgroups) | Tension headache: chronic form |
| 2.3 Headache of tension-type not fulfilling above criteria | Temporomandibular pain and dysfunction syndrome |
| | Osteoarthritis temporomandibular joint (TMJ) |
| | Rheumatoid arthritis of the TMJ |
| | Dystonic disorders |
| | Crushing injury of head or face |
| 3. Cluster headache (more subgroups) | Group V continued: |
| Chronic paroxysmal hemicrania | Cluster headache |
| Cluster headache-like disorder not fulfilling criteria | Chronic paroxysmal hemicrania |
| | Hemicrania continua |
| | Cluster-tic syndrome |
| | Syndrome of 'jabs and jolts' |
| 4. Miscellaneous headaches unassociated with structural lesions (more subgroups) | Headache associated with low CSF pressure Post-dural headache |
| 5. Headache associated with head trauma (more subgroups) | Group V continued: post-traumatic headache |
| 6. Headache associated with vascular disorders (more subgroups) | Group V continued: temporal arthritis, carotidynia |
| 7. Headache associated with non-vascular disorder (more subgroups) | |
| 8. Headache associated with substances or their withdrawal (more subgroups) | |
| 9. Headache associated with non-cephalic infection (more subgroups) | |

## Table 3.1: Continued

| IHS classification | IASP classification |
|---|---|
| 10. Headache associated with metabolic disorders (more subgroups) | |
| 11. Headache or facial pain associated with disorder of cranium, neck, eyes, ears, nose, sinuses, teeth, mouth or other facial or cranial structures | Group IV: lesions of the ear, nose and oral cavity |
| 11.1 Cranial bone | Maxillary sinusitis |
| 11.2 Neck | Odontalgia |
| 11.3 Eyes | Glossodynia and sore mouth |
| 11.4 Ears | Cracked tooth syndrome |
| 11.5 Nose and sinuses | Dry socket |
| 11.6 Teeth, jaws and related structures | Gingival disease |
| 11.7 Temporomandibular joint | Toothache of unknown cause |
| | Inflammatory jaw conditions |
| | Unspecified pain of the jaws |
| | Frostbite of face |
| | Group VII: suboccipital and cervical musculoskeletal disorders |
| 12. Cranial neuralgias, nerve trunk pain and deafferentation pain | Group II: neuralgias of the head and face |
| 12.1 Persistent pain of cranial nerve origin | Trigeminal neuralgia |
| 12.2 Trigeminal neuralgia | Secondary neuralgia (trigeminal) from CNS |
| 12.3 Glossopharyngeal neuralgia | Secondary neuralgia (trigeminal) from trauma |
| 12.4 Nervus intermedius neuralgia | Acute herpes zoster (trigeminal) |
| 12.5 Superior laryngeal neuralgia | Postherpetic neuralgia |
| 12.6 Occipital neuralgia | Geniculate neuralgia |
| 12.7 Central causes of head and facial pain other than tic douloureux | Neuralgia of nervus intermedius |
| 12.8 Pain not fulfilling 11 or 12 | Glossopharyngeal neuralgia (+ from trauma) |
| | Neuralgia of superior laryngeal nerve |
| | Occipital neuralgia |
| | Hypoglossal neuralgia (+ from trauma) |
| | Tolosa–Hunt syndrome |
| | Shortlasting, unilateral neuralgiform pain with conjunctival injection and tearing |
| | Raeder's syndrome |
| 13. Headache not classifiable | Group V continued: headache not otherwise specified |

This broader perspective is a more inclusive method of interpreting the patient's condition. Others have described mechanisms that can produce central sensitization through neural plasticity, and tried to explain the phenomenon of hyperalgesia and how pain can persist (Ren and Dubner, 1999; Sessle, 2000).

Overlap between conditions is greater than might appear from current texts on classification. Many patients who could readily be classified into one defined group have additional features, such as neuropathic, myofascial, migrainous or supra-spinal characteristics (Eide and Rabben, 1998; Graff-Radford, 2000; Sessle, 2000). A classification that accommodates these variant features might lead to a better understanding of the mechanisms involved and also to a better treatment strategy. The IHS (Headache Classification Committee of the IHS, 1988) classification tried to cater for this by allowing for a patient to have more than one disorder, placed in order of importance. However, this does not allow the addition of other 'characteristics' as opposed to an additional diagnosis, which might also help in the patient's management as there are large areas of overlap between most patients' symptoms and their response to treatment. For example, separating headaches from facial pain is an artificial division as many conditions involve both the head and face.

Where facial pain is difficult to classify, it is useful to try and break it down into a combination of elements, be it neuropathic, myofascial, migrainous or supraspinous (*Table 3.2*), rather than calling it 'unclassifiable'. Nevertheless, these terms do not allow those who have previously escaped classification to be neatly categorized, as these patients often have features of more than one type of pain.

## Diagnosis

It is essential to take a structured history to reach the correct diagnosis, plan the right treatment and avoid misguided interventions that only complicate the picture. It might be thought that a completely different subgroup of patients will present to each specialty — this is not the case. Most people know that their sinuses lie behind the facial bones, so many conclude that the cause of their facial pain lies in their sinuses before they seek medical help. 'Sinus trouble' is an acceptable label in the community, while atypical facial pain or 'unclassifiable pain' are not. However, rhinosinusitis rarely causes facial pain, even in an ear, nose and throat clinic (see later). Many patients label themselves as having sinusitis when this is not the case.

Facial pain has a special emotional significance: symptom interpretation is often influenced by cognitive, affective and motivational factors. For a few patients, facial pain may be the channel by which they express emotional distress, anxiety or the psychological harm associated with disease, trauma or surgery. It may be the means by which they demand attention or obtain secondary gain. The presence of a marked psychological overlay does not mean that there is no underlying organic problem, but it should make one wary about invasive treatment. If there is a big discrepancy between the patient's affect and the description of the pain, the organic component of the illness may be of relatively minor importance.

## Table 3.2: The main types of pain

| Characteristics | Migrainous | Myofascial | Neuropathic | Supraspinal |
|---|---|---|---|---|
| Poorly localized | | +++ | + | ++ |
| Continuous dysaesthesia | | | +++ | + |
| Fluctuating duration and intensity | | +++ | | ++ |
| Location varies | | ++ | | ++ |
| Pressure, tight, ache | | +++ | | |
| Burning | | | +++ | ++ |
| Electric, sharp | | | +++ | + |
| Sensation of numbness, swelling | | ++ | ++ | ++ |
| History of injury | | | +++ | + |
| Phantom pain | | | +++ | + |
| Nausea | +++ | | + if severe pain | |
| Aura/photophobia | Classical | | | |
| More common in women/ hormonal factors | ++ | ++ | ++ | ++ |
| Age | | | Increased incidence | |
| Psychological stress/ emotional conflict | | ++ | + | ++ |
| Hyperaesthesia of skin | | ++ | ++ | |
| Hyperaesthesia of muscles | | +++ | ++ | |
| Hyperaemia, erythema | +++ | ++ | ++ | + |
| Response to neural blockade | | ++ | Peripheral neuropathic pain | Can get placebo effect |
| Responds to behavioural therapy | | ++ | + | ++ |
| Responds to tricyclic antidepressants | + | + relaxation/ biofeedback | ++ | ++ |

Pain that remains constant for many months or years or which extends either across the midline or across defined dermatomes is less likely to have a physical basis. However, pain associated with clear exacerbating or relieving factors, whose onset was clear-cut and whose site does not vary during the consultation, usually has an organic cause. Should the diagnosis remain obscure, re-taking the history at the next consultation may be helpful, or a symptom diary kept by the patient may help.

A careful history is central to a correct diagnosis. Twelve questions form the basis of an algorithm that will help reach a differential diagnosis.

### 1. Where is the pain and does it radiate anywhere?

Asking the patient to point with one finger to the site of the pain is helpful, not only because it localizes the pain but also because the gesture made often relays information about its nature (e.g. patients with myofascial pain give a vague gesture over a broad area; with neuropathic pain, such as post-traumatic neuralgia or trigeminal neuralgia, it is well localized), and the facial expression indicates its emotional significance to the patient.

### 2. Is it deep or superficial?

Deep pain is dull and poorly localized, but pain from the skin tends to be sharp and well defined.

### 3. Is the pain continuous or intermittent?

The periodicity of symptoms may be a pointer to the diagnosis, such as being woken in the early hours by severe facial pain that lasts up to 2 hours suggests cluster headache.

### 4. How did the pain begin?

An aura preceding unilateral facial pain or headache is typical of classical migraine.

### 5. How often does the pain occur?

Recurrent bouts of aching of the ear and jaw with sharp twinges is a pattern characteristic of temporomandibular joint (TMJ) dysfunction, while monthly premenstrual headaches with nausea are typical of migraine.

### 6. What is the pattern of the attacks and are they progressing?

The relentless progression of a headache, in particular if associated with nausea or effortless vomiting, is worrying, and an intracranial lesion should be sought.

### 7. How long is each episode?

The stabbing pain of trigeminal neuralgia is short lived with a refractory period.

### 8. What precipitates the pain?

Trigeminal neuralgia is initiated by a specific trigger point.

### 9. What relieves the pain?

Tension headaches do not respond to analgesics, whereas patients with migraine often report that lying quietly in a dark room helps.

**10. Are there any associated symptoms?**
If nausea accompanies the pain, this is characteristic, although not diagnostic, of migraine.

**11. How does it affect daily life and sleep?**
Should the patient describe a severe unrelenting pain but have an apparently normal life and pattern of sleep, atypical facial pain should be considered in the differential diagnosis.

**12. What treatment has been tried and with what effect?**
Tension headache and atypical facial pain fail to respond to analgesics; this in isolation does not clinch the diagnosis but is a useful pointer. Chronic paroxysmal hemicrania specifically responds to indomethacin, and trigeminal neuralgia to carbamazepine.

# Types of facial pain

The following are brief descriptions of the common types of facial pain, with or without headache, in the order used by the IHS classification, omitting groups with headache alone.

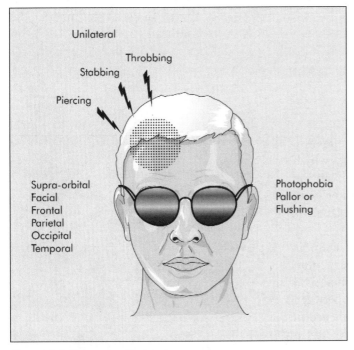

*Figure 3.1: Features of migraine.*

### Migraine

Migraine primarily causes severe headache, but in a small proportion of patients it can affect the cheek, orbit and forehead. Migraine is a term that is often wrongly used by patients, and the diagnosis needs confirmation by precise questioning. Classical migraine with an aura and visual disturbances rarely affects the face (*Figure 3.1*).

Common migraine, nine times more frequent, is described as sharp, severe and pulsatile in nature and is invariably accompanied by nausea. There is, however, no premonition or photopsia. Stress, diet, premenstrual state and barometric changes can induce it, and it is worth asking about these and other trigger factors. There is often a family history of migraine.

27

## Tension-type headache

Tension-type headache is described as a feeling of tightness, pressure or constriction that varies in intensity, frequency and duration. It usually affects the forehead or temple and often has a suboccipital component (*Figure 3.2*).

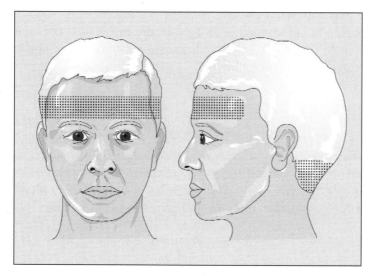

Figure 3.2: Localization of tension-type headache.

It may be episodic or chronic (>15 days/month, >6 months) and is only occasionally helped by non-steroidal anti-inflammatory drugs (NSAIDs). Typically, patients are taking large quantities of analgesics of all kinds, but say that they have little benefit (Olesen, 1991). It is often associated with anxiety, depression or agitated depression. Hyperaesthesia of the skin or muscles of the forehead often occurs, causing the patient to think they have rhinosinusitis, as they know their sinuses lie under the forehead.

## Cluster headache

This typically presents with a severe, unilateral, stabbing or burning pain, which may be frontal, temporal, ocular, over the cheek or even in the maxillary teeth (*Figure 3.3*). Pain is therefore facial, and 'headache' is a misnomer.

Nausea is absent but frequently there is rhinorrhoea, unilateral nasal obstruction, lacrimation and sometimes conjunctival infection. It is most common in men between 20–40 years of age. The patient is awakened in the early hours, often walking around in distress, with the pain lasting between 30 minutes–2 hours. It may be precipitated by alcohol intake. Myosis or facial flushing may be seen.

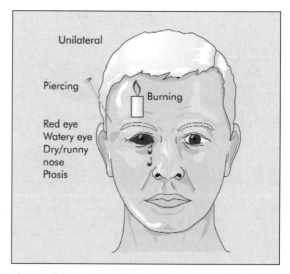

Figure 3.3: Features of cluster headache.

## Chronic paroxysmal hemicrania

Chronic paroxysmal hemicrania is an excruciating pain occurring in women at any time of night or day. It can affect the frontal, ocular, cheek or temporal regions and last 30 minutes–3 hours. The patient can experience several episodes in 24 hours, and nasal congestion, lacrimation and facial flushing can all be a feature.

## Associated pains

These include headache or facial pain associated with disorders of the cranium, neck, eyes, ears, nose, sinuses, teeth, mouth or other facial or cranial structures.

## Eyes

Uncorrected optical refractive errors can cause headaches, but their importance is exaggerated. Optic nerve disease results in reduced acuity and colour vision. Pain on ocular movement suggests optic neuritis or scleritis. It is vital to recognize acute glaucoma, which may cause severe orbital pain and headache. The patient may see haloes around lights, and circumcorneal injection can occur as well as systemic upset, especially vomiting. This requires urgent treatment, as vision is rapidly lost.

Pain is a feature of periorbital cellulitis, which may present with lid swelling and erythema if it is preseptal, and with chemosis and proptosis.

Orbital pain can also be caused by uveitis, keratitis, dry eye syndrome and convergence insufficiency.

## Ears

Earache without any hearing loss and with a normal eardrum is usually caused by referred pain from the TMJ, tonsil, tongue base or hypopharynx. These should be examined.

## Nose and sinuses

Patients not infrequently complain of 'sinus', believing that they have sinusitis. This often used term should be treated with scepticism. Acute infective sinusitis causes severe pain that is usually well localized over the affected sinus, follows an upper respiratory tract infection, and the patient has a temperature. However, chronic sinusitis is often painless, causing nasal obstruction as a result of mucosal hypertrophy and a purulent discharge throughout the day (not just a collection in the morning that is usually the result of postnasal mucus stagnating in a mouthbreather or snorer that has become discoloured by local commensals).

An acute exacerbation can cause pain, but this rarely lasts more than a few days. Symptoms of a dull ache behind the eyes, affecting the lower part of the forehead, under the nasal bridge or either side of the nose are often not related to sinus disease and are caused by an extension of tension-type headache. The term used to describe this is midfacial segment pain, and it is described later as it is not in the IHS classification.

Facial pain without any nasal symptoms is unlikely to be caused by sinusitis.

## Imaging

Plain X-rays have a poor specificity and sensitivity in sinusitis management. Computed tomography (CT) is not much better, as about 30% of asymptomatic people have false–positive changes in one or more of their sinuses on CT scanning (Bhattachayya et al, 1997; Jones et al, 1997). Rigid endoscopy provides more accurate information about the extent of sinus disease. However, patients with facial pain who have no objective evidence of sinus disease (endoscopy and CT negative) and whose pain does not respond to medical antibiotic or steroid therapy aimed at treating sinonasal disease are unlikely to be helped by surgery for more than a few months (Acquadro et al, 1997; Ruoff, 1997; Tarabichi, 2000; West and Jones, 2001). It seems that surgery can alter central neuronal activity in one-third of these patients for up to 12 months, but in one-third the pain is worse and in the remaining third there is no difference.

Previous theories implicating contact points as a cause of facial pain have been discredited, as they are found as frequently in an asymptomatic population as in those with pain, and these patients often respond to low-dose amitriptyline.

Plain sinus radiographs have no role in diagnosing chronic rhinosinusitis.

CT scans show changes in 30% of asymptomatic individuals.

Occasionally, following a nasal fracture, pain or paraesthesiae can persist over the nasal bridge. The cause of this is unclear; it may be the result of a neuroma in the scar tissue, but seems to be influenced by the degree of distress the patient continues to feel about the insult he or she has received. Why some people develop neuropathic pain after an injury while others do not may centre on whether central neural plasticity occurs to inhibit peripheral neural changes that might otherwise lead to dysaesthesia, hyperaesthesia or chronic pain instead of central sensitization or downregulation of central inhibition (Ren and Dubner, 1999; Sessle, 2000). Peripheral regenerative or deafferent changes may influence the trigeminal brainstem sensory nuclear complex, just as nerve compression, sympathetically-mediated pain and neuroma formation can cause neuropathic pain.

## Other diseases of the nose or sinuses

Carcinoma of the maxilla is rare. Patients unfortunately often present late when the disease has spread beyond the confines of the sinus. Unilateral, bloody, purulent nasal discharge is the most frequent presentation. Less common symptoms are infraorbital paraesthesiae, loose teeth or ill-fitting dentures, proptosis, deformity of the cheek, nasal obstruction or epistaxis. Pain is a late feature.

Nasopharyngeal carcinoma is also rare but presents most commonly in young adults from the Far East. It often presents with cervical lymphadenopathy and middle-ear effusions. However, its spread can involve the fifth and sixth cranial nerves, causing facial pain or a lateral rectus palsy.

Tolosa–Hunt syndrome (recurrent painful ophthalmoplegia) occurs equally in both sexes at any age. It presents with gnawing unilateral orbital pain with relapsing and remitting paralysis of the third, fourth and sixth cranial nerves. Occasionally, there is paraesthesia of the forehead. It is caused by a lesion in the region of the cavernous sinus or the superior orbital fissure. It should be differentiated from ophthalmoplegic migraine, painful diabetic oculomotor palsy and malignancy. Although the condition often responds to steroids, this is not diagnostic.

Raeder's paratrigeminal syndrome presents as an intense, sharp pain or ache around the ophthalmic division of the trigeminal cranial nerve, with associated myosis, ptosis and facial hypoaesthesia in the same area. The corneal reflex is reduced, but there is no reduced sweating as in Horner's syndrome. A lesion near the base of the middle cranial fossa at the medial border of the Gasserian ganglion is responsible, caused by a carotid aneurysm, metastasis or local neoplastic invasion.

### Teeth, jaws and related structures

Afferent fibres from the dental pulp, being small and unmyelinated, produce poorly localized pain, which often radiates to surrounding structures but rarely crosses the midline. However, dentino-enamel defects produce a sharp, usually well-localized, excruciating pain, often followed by a dull ache. This may be caused by cervical erosion or a lost or cracked filling, and induced by temperature change, osmotic or mechanical stimuli.

Pain becomes more localized once the periodontium is involved. The periodontium may be affected either by the formation of a periapical abscess involving the periodontium at the tooth's apex, or by infection in a pocket around the tooth where there has been long-standing gingival and periodontal inflammation. Acute pulpitis causes a dull ache with exacerbations of excruciating pain, and often radiates or is referred to the adjacent ipsilateral jaw. Chronic pulpitis causes a dull, difficult-to-define ache, which may be worse when lying flat. Clinical examination usually reveals a carious tooth or leaking restoration, and toothache is initiated or exacerbated by hot and cold stimuli.

'Phantom tooth pain' is said to follow a dental extraction with incomplete osseous repair. Necrotic bone and neural elements have been found in some patients with this syndrome, but in most it is a form of atypical facial pain (see later). All too often the pain precedes the extraction, which has been done in part through pressure from patients' belief that their pain is dental when it was a form of atypical facial pain.

### Temporomandibular joint dysfunction

Temporomandibular joint dysfunction is most commonly unilateral (90%), and usually occurs in young adults with a history of bruxism, clenching, trauma, recent dental work, anxiety, enthusiastic kissing or cradling the telephone between the jaw and the shoulder. Another contributing factor is poor occlusion, as occurs in crossbite, or in a partially edentulous patient without an appropriate denture, or in someone with a completely edentulous mouth whose dentures are worn or have been made with an inadequate vertical height resulting in overclosure.

Pain is caused by pterygoid spasm and is described as a deep, dull ache that may masquerade as toothache or earache. There is often a superimposed sharper component that may radiate down the jaw or over the side of the face or temple (*Figure 3.4*).

It is often necessary to ask whether chewing exacerbates symptoms, as this is rarely volunteered. Spasm may be initiated by a reflex mechanism to avoid an undesirable pattern of malocclusion. Anxiety lowers the threshold for this mechanism, and it often occurs in people under stress. Clicking of the TMJ is an

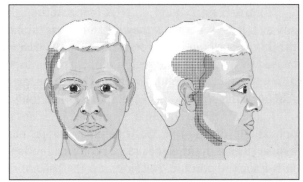

*Figure 3.4: Distribution of pain in temporomandibular joint dysfunction.*

unreliable sign, whereas pain on palpation of the insertion of the lateral pterygoid is a better indicator. This can be demonstrated with the gloved little finger where the lateral pterygoid muscle can be palpated at the most posterior end of the upper buccal sulcus. Trismus and deviation of the jaw from the midline on opening, as well as evidence of malocclusion or a high shiny spot on a filling, should be sought. Radiographs are normally of little help in making the diagnosis, but may show degenerative changes in rheumatoid arthritis or gout where there is a suspicion of an arthropathy.

Eagle's syndrome produces pain that may be felt in the lateral wall of the pharynx, the mandible, the floor of the mouth or the side of the neck. A nagging discomfort lasting seconds to minutes is precipitated on opening the mouth or head turning. An elongated styloid process with a calcified stylohyoid ligament may be palpated laterally or via the tonsillar fossa, and can be seen on an oblique radiograph.

Glossodynia is characterized by a burning sensation in the tongue, and there is often disordered taste or the sensation of a dry mouth. The oral cavity should be inspected for signs of ulceration or erythroplakia, and the cause of these investigated and treated. Local irritation, lichen planus, diabetes mellitus, candida, serum iron deficiency, vitamin B12 deficiency, irritant mouthwashes, a drug reaction, denture component sensitivity and galvanism should be excluded. In some patients, no cause can be found and this group is over-represented by women over 50 years old, often with a cancer phobia, a history of an emotional disturbance or a precipitating major life event.

### Cranial neuralgias, nerve trunk pain and deafferentation pain

Trigeminal neuralgia is more common in women over 40 years of age with a peak incidence between 50–60 years. Patients complain of paroxysms of agonizing lancinating pain, induced by a specific trigger point. Repetitive bursts can be triggered usually with a refractory period of more than

30 seconds. In more than a third of sufferers, the pain occurs in both the maxillary and mandibular divisions, while in a fifth it is confined to the mandibular region and in 3% to the ophthalmic division. A sufferer can always localize the trigger zone but is reluctant to demonstrate it.

Typical trigger sites are the lips and nasolabial folds, but touching the gingivae may also trigger pain. Some patients report that firm pressure over the trigger point helps and delays a further bout. A flush may be seen over the area in question, but there are no sensory disturbances in primary trigeminal neuralgia. Remissions are common, but it is not unusual for attacks to increase in frequency and severity. Histology shows proliferative and disorganized changes in the myelin sheath of the nerve involved. Janetta (1976) found that a percentage had vascular compression of the trigeminal nerve. However, this has been noted in many normal cadavers. Beware the dental pain that can mimic trigeminal neuralgia, particularly a fractured tooth or exposed cervical dentine. Secondary trigeminal neuralgia is attributable to a discernible pathological cause. In patients under 40 years old, it is most commonly caused by multiple sclerosis, while over this age a tumour, aneurysm or meningioma can cause the pain.

Postherpetic neuralgia affects an eighth of patients suffering from herpes zoster infection. Thankfully, two-thirds of these recover in the first year. It is more common in the elderly, and if it persists for more than a year it is unlikely to resolve. It causes a persistent, intense burning or lancinating pain, and where there is a sensory loss there is more likely to be associated dysaesthesia. Patients often become depressed and irritable. Histology shows demyelination together with a disproportionate loss of large nerve fibres, and this may allow increased transmission in nocioceptive fibres through the dorsal horn, thus causing pain. Zoster appears to have some effect at the suprathalamic level, as tractotomy at a more peripheral level is of little help.

Mental nerve neuralgia can mimic trigeminal neuralgia by producing sharp pain in the lower lip and chin, when the lower premolar area is touched in the edentulous patient. It is the result of exposure and irritation of the mental nerve branch of the inferior alveolar nerve in a long-standing edentulous patient whose alveolar bone has atrophied. Direct pressure from either a denture or finger can initiate this unpleasant sharp pain.

### Glossopharyngeal neuralgia

Glossopharyngeal neuralgia is rare, being 100 times less common than trigeminal neuralgia. A stabbing pain is felt in the tonsillar region and ipsilateral ear (rarely in the base of the tongue and angle of the jaw). It is precipitated by swallowing or talking, and bouts last for weeks or months, with a tendency to recur.

### Other causes of persistent pain of cranial nerve origin

Stretching the arterial tree, which supplies the proximal portions of the cranial nerves and the dura within 1 cm of any venous sinus, induces a headache but can also cause facial pain. The supratentorial vessels and dura refer pain to the ophthalmic division of the trigeminal nerve. Infratentorial structures refer pain to the distribution of the glossopharyngeal and vagus nerve and the upper three cervical nerve dermatomes. Space-occupying lesions, e.g. meningiomas, angiomas and intracerebral metastases, can induce facial pain by irritation of the trigeminal nerve along its intracerebral course.

*Facial pain not fulfilling groups of 'headaches and facial pain involving the head and neck'
or 'cranial neuralgias, nerve trunk pain and deafferentation pain'*

### *'Atypical facial pain, atypical odontalgia'*

Atypical facial pain is not a dustbin term, and it has many distinguishing features that make it a diagnosis in its own right, not one to resort to in despair. It should only be made reluctantly when organic causes have been excluded. It is often complicated by surgical procedures, which have been performed in an attempt to alleviate symptoms that have been misdiagnosed.

The description of symptoms often does not correlate with the patient's affect; there can be unusual associated factors, exaggerated responses to the pain and often psychological factors or an excess of unpleasant life events. While psychological factors are always important in any patient's interpretation of facial pain, in this condition they play an overwhelming role. Pain is typically deep and ill-defined, changes location, is unexplainable on an anatomical basis, occurs almost daily and is sometimes fluctuating, sometimes continuous, without any precipitating factors and is not relieved by analgesics. Often more specific questioning about symptoms results in increasingly vague answers. The pain does not wake the patient up, and while the patient reports that they cannot sleep, they often look well rested. It is more common in women over the age of 40 years, and typically lasts many months. A proportion has symptoms of depressive illness or anxiety neurosis, or has problems adjusting to the difficulties that life presents. Some patients appear to be so used to their pain that its loss would force them to dramatically reappraise their life. Confrontation is counterproductive, while sympathetic discussion, close liaison with the GP and possibly psychiatric help may be beneficial. Tricyclic antidepressants are often of help, in particular when there are symptoms of endogenous depression, e.g. loss of appetite and interest in life, self-neglect, early morning waking and fatigue.

The description of hysterical pain is often vague with unusual neurological symptoms, such as weakness and paraesthesia. No physical lesion can be found and the distribution of neurological loss does not conform to the known anatomy. Pain occurs throughout the day, although fluctuating in severity. It enables the patient to obtain some personal benefit, often by avoiding an unwanted task.

## Non-classifiable facial pain

Although not in the IHS classification, pain can be characterized as to whether it has neuropathic, myofascial, migrainous or supraspinal features.

A further group of patients whose symptoms have evaded classification to date are those with symmetrical facial (with or without forehead) pain, which has all the same characteristics as tension-type headache but a different distribution of pain (*Figures 3.5a–h*).

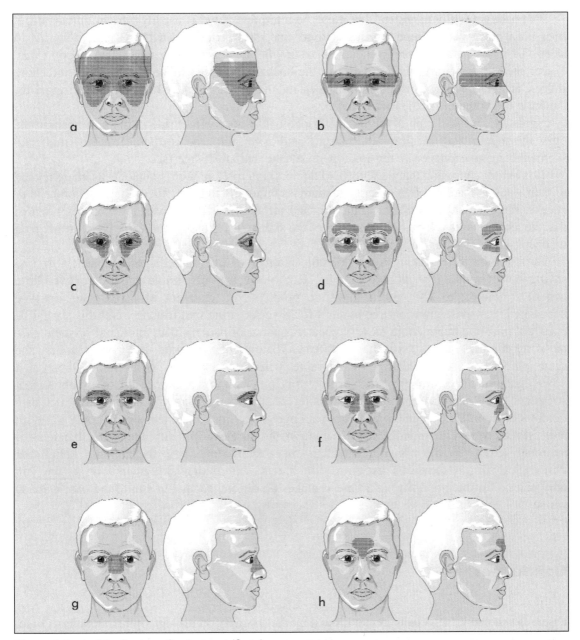

*Figure 3.5a–h: Distribution of pain in midfacial segment pain.*

'Midfacial segment pain' avoids the use of the term 'tension' used in 'tension-type' headache, and avoids the confusion that this term causes the patient. The pain usually affects the nasal area, around or behind the eyes or the cheeks, and not uncommonly involves the forehead. It is described as a pressing or aching pain, similar to the feeling of constriction or tightening. It can affect each area in isolation or in combination, but it is usually symmetrical unless there has been trauma or surgery to one side, when the features of atypical facial pain can be superimposed on a background of midfacial segment pain.

The pain is usually persistent, but it can be intermittent and is usually present on waking. It does not worsen with routine physical activity and rarely interferes with the patient getting to sleep. To make matters more complex, the stimulus of a genuine acute sinus infection may exacerbate the symptoms, with a return to the background faceache on resolution of infection. Indeed, an episode of acute rhinosinusitis occasionally appears to have been the initial trigger for the onset of symptoms in the first instance.

Symmetrical facial pain involving the bridge of the nose, either side of the nose, behind the eyes, the supraorbital or infraorbital margins and/or the forehead is often caused by midfacial segment pain, an extension of tension-type headache that affects the face.

It is hardly surprising that patients (and doctors) interpret all their symptoms as being related to their sinuses. Patients often describe tenderness on lightly touching the skin of the forehead or cheeks, along with hyperaesthesia of the skin and soft tissues in these areas. It is important to note that the tenderness is felt on light touching of the skin and soft tissue, and there is no further pain on deep palpation of the underlying bone.

Sufferers are often taking a considerable number of over-the-counter analgesics, despite saying they help little if at all. In the author's experience, the only simple analgesic of even little benefit is ibuprofen. The current first-line prophylactic treatment of chronic tension-type headache is low-dose amitriptyline at night for 6 weeks in the first instance, and this should be tried as a first-line treatment in these patients. A quarter of patients with midfacial segment pain have migrainous features associated with exacerbations of their pain, and approximately the same proportion have a history of migraine. There is also a suggestion that there is a downregulation of central inhibition from supraspinal impulses as a result of psychological stress and emotional disturbances. It is of interest that if surgery is mistakenly performed as a treatment for midfacial segment pain, the pain may sometimes abate temporarily, only to return after several weeks to months. It is as though the surgical stimulus alters the 'balance' of neuronal activity in the trigeminal nucleus for a short time. It is the author's belief that rhinological surgery should be discouraged in patients with midfacial segment pain, as the pain only helps a third temporarily; in a third it makes no difference, and in a third the pain is made worse.

## Conclusions

Diseases that cause facial pain are not limited by the specialty on the sign of the outpatient clinic, and it is therefore absolutely essential to be aware of the alternative diagnoses.

## References

Acquadro MA, Salman SD, Joseph MP (1997) Analysis of pain and endoscopic sinus surgery for sinusitis. *Ann Otol Rhinol Laryngol* **106**: 30–9

Bendtsen L (2000) Central sensitization in tension-type headache – possible pathophysiological mechanisms. *Cephalalgia* **20**: 486–508

Bendtsen L, Jensen R, Olesen J (1996) Qualitatively altered nociception in chronic myofascial pain. *Pain* **65**: 259–64

Bhattachayya T, Piccirillo J, Wippold FJ (1997) Relationship between patient-based descriptions of sinusitis and paranasal sinus computed tomographic findings. *Arch Otolaryngol Head Neck Surg* **123**: 1189–92

Eide PK, Rabben T (1998) Trigeminal neuropathic pain: pathophysiological mechanisms examined by quantitative assessment of abnormal pain and sensory perception. *Neurosurgery* **43**: 1103–9

Graff-Radford SB (2000) Facial pain. *Curr Opin Neurol* **13**: 291–6

Headache Classification Committee of the International Headache Society (1988) Classification and diagnostic criteria for headache disorders, cranial neuralgias and facial pain. *Cephalalgia* **8** (Suppl 7): 1–93

International Association for the Study of Pain (1994) In: Merskey H, Bogduk N, eds. *Classification of Chronic Pain.* IAPS Press, Seattle: 59–95

Janetta PJ (1976) Microsurgical approach to the trigeminal nerve for tic douloureux. *Prog Neurol Surg* **7**: 180–200

Jensen R (1999) Pathophysiological mechanisms of tension-type headache: a review of epidemiological and experimental studies. *Cephalalgia* **19**: 602–21

Jensen R, Olesen J (2000) Tension-type headache: an update on mechanisms and treatment. *Curr Opin Neurol* **13**: 285–9

Jones NS, Strobl A, Holland I (1997) CT findings in 100 patients with rhinosinusitis and 100 controls. *Clin Otolaryngol* **22**: 47–51

Olesen J (1991) Clinical and pathophysiological observations in migraine and tension-type headache explained by integration of vascular, supraspinal and myofascial inputs. *Pain* **46**: 125–32

Olesen J, Rasmussen BK (1995) Classification of primary headaches. *Biomedicine Pharmacother* **49**: 446–51

Ren K, Dubner R (1999) Central nervous system plasticity and persistent pain. *J Orofacial Pain* **13**: 155–63

Ruoff GE (1997) When sinus headache isn't sinus headache. *Headache Q* **8**: 22–31

Sessle BJ (2000) Acute and chronic craniofacial pain: brainstem mechanisms and nociceptive transmission and neuroplasticity, and their clinical correlates. *Crit Rev Oral Biol Med* **11**(1): 57–91

Tarabichi M (2000) Characteristics of sinus-related pain. *Otolaryngol Head Neck Surg* **122**: 84–7

West B, Jones NS (2001) Endoscopy-negative, computed tomography-negative facial pain in a nasal clinic. *Laryngoscope* **111**(4 pt 1): 581–6

# Chapter 4

# Modern management of migraine

*Giles Elrington*

Migraine presents with episodic disabling headache, with additional features that distinguish it from other headache syndromes: it is not 'just a headache'. Treatment must be carefully selected, titrated and adjusted according to individual patient response.

Migraine affects one in ten people. It is diagnosed from the patient's history: examination is normal, and investigation usually unnecessary. Treatments include acute rescue, lifestyle strategies, alternative remedies and prophylactic drugs. Most patients are managed in primary care; many never consult a doctor. The triptans have improved acute treatment and renewed scientific interest in migraine. Overuse of acute rescue medication can cause chronic daily headache.

## Pathophysiology

Migraine reflects spontaneous overactivity and abnormal amplification in pain and other pathways originating in the brainstem. Goadsby's (2001) review of current opinion favours a primarily neural cause, exacerbated by feedback loops involving cranial arteries in the trigeminovascular system. A relative deficiency of 5-hydroxytriptamine (5-HT) may be near the root cause, and explains the action of most drug treatments. The relevance of calcium channel abnormalities is being studied, and peptides such as calcitonin gene-related peptide, which may be closer than 5-HT to the underlying cause, offer hope for improved treatment in the future. Migraine may be inherited via multiple genes. Some rare migraine variants, such as familial hemiplegic migraine, are single gene disorders. These may be neurodegenerative rather than headache disorders.

## Differential diagnosis

Migraine is typically manifest by episodic disabling headache, although it is more than just head pain. Differential diagnosis is from tension-type headache (TTH), with which migraine is comorbid, probably on a spectrum rather than as a distinct disease. Migraine lasts hours or days, is absent more often than is present, and the average attack frequency is once a month. TTH is often chronic, and is present more often than is absent. Migraine and TTH should be distinguished from cluster headache, which is relatively rare and causes recurrent, daily headache that is unilateral with autonomic dysfunction. The third common, although often challenging, differential diagnosis is medication-overuse headache (MOH). This typically complicates migraine, which is transformed into a chronic, daily headache similar to chronic TTH.

# Diagnosis

The International Headache Society (IHS) criteria (1988), abbreviated in *Table 4.1*, are invaluable in diagnosing migraine. These may be too restrictive, and can be interpreted flexibly by experienced clinicians. There are two main types of migraine: migraine without aura and migraine with aura. Many people have both; migraine without aura is at least three times as common as migraine with aura. Family history, trigger factors and treatment response have no diagnostic value.

### Migraine without aura

This was formerly called common migraine. A diagnosis of migraine without aura is suggested by a history of episodic headache lasting at least a few hours and at most a few days, accompanied by gastrointestinal symptoms or by oversensitive special senses. IHS criteria may be fulfilled when pain is mild or generalized: it does not have to be severe or unilateral. Migraine is disabling. It is unusual to be able distract oneself from migraine without aura with exercise or hard work. The IHS criteria do not emphasize the periodicity of migraine: a person who describes a migraine attack more than twice every week is unlikely to have migraine without aura alone, although may have migraine without aura complicated by MOH and/or TTH. This is common in patients referred with 'intractable migraine' or 'status migrainosus'.

### Migraine with aura

This used to be called focal or classical migraine. Visual aura is often so characteristic that migraine with aura is easily diagnosed. Auras affecting sensation, movement, cognition, vestibular function or consciousness may be worrying, and are occasionally difficult to distinguish from thromboembolism or from epilepsy (especially occipital seizures). New migraine with aura is often associated with a longer history of migraine without aura, mistakenly diagnosed as 'bilious attacks', 'sinusitis' or 'normal headaches'. Migraine aura evolves over time, usually many minutes; one aspect of aura improves while another is deteriorating. Visual symptoms are positive (seeing things that are not there), homonymous and binocular. Aura typically precedes migraine headache, although it can occur at any time in relation to pain.

**Table 4.1: Abbreviated International Headache Society (1988) criteria for the common primary headaches**

| Type of headache | Criteria | |
| --- | --- | --- |
| Migraine without aura | Headache lasting 4 hours–3 days | |
| | Nausea/vomiting and/or light and noise sensitivity | |
| | Two of the following | Unilateral pain |
| | | Moderate- or severe-intensity pain |
| | | Aggravation by simple physical activity |
| | | Pulsating pain |
| Migraine with aura | At least three of the following | Reversible brainstem or cortical dysfunction |
| | | Aura develops over >4 minutes, or 2 auras in succession |
| | | Each aura <60 minutes |
| | | Headache <60 minutes following aura |
| Episodic tension-type headache | Duration 30 minutes–7 days | |
| | At least two of the following | Mild- or moderate-intensity pain |
| | | Bilateral pain |
| | | No aggravation by simple physical activity |
| | | Pressing or tight (non-pulsating) pain |
| | No nausea/vomiting; may have light or noise sensitivity (not both) | |
| Chronic tension-type headache | >15 days pain per month, for >6 months | |
| | At least two of the following | Mild- or moderate-intensity pain |
| | | Bilateral pain |
| | | No aggravation by simple physical activity |
| | | Pressing or tight (non-pulsating) pain |
| | No vomiting; one only of nausea, light sensitivity, noise sensitivity | |
| Cluster headache | Severe unilateral peri-orbital pain lasting 15–180 minutes | |
| | Pain frequency alternate days, to eight per day | |
| | Autonomic dysfunction, ipsilateral to and accompanying pain | |

All of the above diagnostic criteria require the exclusion of secondary (i.e. structural) causes for pain. This is normally achieved on clinical grounds

Aura is not always contralateral to pain. Migraine aura without headache is common. Thromboembolism may be accompanied by headache (especially with vertebral or carotid dissection, in which pain usually precedes impairment), but is distinguished from migraine with aura by abrupt, non-evolving associated impairment, confined to a single vascular territory.

## History

The patient should be encouraged to give a spontaneous account of his or her symptoms. Specific enquiry should establish the duration and frequency of pain. Associated symptoms should be sought: many who deny nausea will readily acknowledge queasiness. Light and noise sensitivity may be denied by a patient who retreats to the dark and quiet. Do not ask about phono- and photophobia, but ask what the patient does during an attack. Many headache sufferers can identify more than one type of attack: ask specifically about this.

Previous and current treatments must be documented. Note drugs, doses and duration: many take ineffective or weak agents, at insufficient dose and at inappropriate times. Overuse of acute medication is common, revealed by careful enquiry. People taking daily combination analgesics or triptans often dissemble: 'I keep it to a minimum'; 'I only use it when the pain is bad'. Treatment response is typically described as 'it takes the edge off it'.

Rather than ask how many tablets are taken each day, establish frequency and quantity of prescription or purchase ('12 extra-strong painkillers, twice a week', '200 co-codamol a month'). The number of medication stashes is often revealing: those who depend upon treatment biochemically or emotionally will store supplies in their handbag or briefcase, bedroom, bathroom, kitchen, office and car.

Treatment response does not define headache: many people with migraine do not respond to 'migraine tablets' (including triptans), and those who report benefit do not necessarily have migraine.

## Examination

Examination is primarily aimed at excluding structural brain lesions. It is also an opportunity to screen for comorbid disease such as hypertension and depression; neither of which commonly cause headaches.

In outpatient practice, the 'full neurological examination' is neither necessary nor possible in the time available. *Table 4.2* lists the author's personal screen, which has been criticized both for its brevity and its length. Ataxia and papilloedema are probably the two most important physical signs.

**Table 4.2: Suggested brief CNS examination for routine, outpatient headache practice**

Romberg's sign

Tandem gait

Drift of outstretched hands

Finger–nose test

Finger dexterity

Binocular visual fields, to confrontation

Eye movements

Facial weakness

Pupillary responses and Horner's syndrome

Tendon reflexes and plantar responses

Fundoscopy

# Investigation

Most people with migraine are managed in primary care and need no investigation. People with possible migraine are investigated to exclude other causes of migraine-like symptoms.

## Imaging

Brain imaging is often considered for people with headache or migraine; Steiner et al (2001) state that imaging is rarely necessary. Imaging may reassure or, conversely, may generate concern. Arguably, every painful head should be imaged. This would result in an impossible workload. Rasmussen and Stewart's survey (2000) shows that 18% of women and 6% of men have migraine; 2–3% have chronic daily headache. If imaged once with normal results, when should imaging be repeated? The author's experience (Elrington, 1997) is that about one-third of UK headache patients in secondary or tertiary care are imaged, two-thirds of which occurs before neurological referral. In practice it can be difficult and unhelpful to resist demand for imaging in a patient-centred healthcare system. Magnetic resonance imaging is always preferable to computed tomography because of better resolution and lack of irradiation. The exception is for emergency presentation with possible cerebral haemorrhage, as fresh blood is better imaged with computed tomography than magnetic resonance imaging. Suggested guidance for the rationing of imaging is given in *Table 4.3*.

## Table 4.3: Brain imaging strategies for headache patients

|  | **Mandatory imaging** |
| --- | --- |
| First, worst, thunderclap headache | Computed tomography (emergency) |
| Exertional, cough or valsalva headache | Magnetic resonance imaging |
| Headache and signs suggesting brain lesion | Magnetic resonance imaging or computed tomography |
| Headache and known malignancy | Magnetic resonance imaging or computed tomography with contrast |
|  | **Optional imaging** |
| New headache in older person | Magnetic resonance imaging or computed tomography |
| Headache, not migraine without aura, migraine with aura, tension-type headache, medication overuse headache or cluster | Magnetic resonance imaging or computed tomography |

### Other tests

People over 60 years of age with new headache should have an erythrocyte sedimentation rate to consider the possibility of giant cell (temporal) arteritis, which is not common in headache practice. A chest X-ray should be considered in smokers, or those who may have metastatic cancer.

## Treatment

Most people with migraine need treatment. Some with infrequent or relatively mild attacks may prefer just to rest while the migraine attack settles naturally. Rest is important for most migraine attacks; sleep, if possible, can abort migraine. It is important to differentiate between acute rescue and prophylactic treatment. Guidelines have been published in the UK (Steiner et al, 2001) and the USA (Silberstein, 2000).

# Acute rescue

## Analgesics and antiemetics

A simple analgesic provides effective relief from many migraines. Absorption is impaired by gastric stasis during migraine; this may be helped by the addition of an antiemetic (even if nausea or vomiting are not prominent), and by use of a large dose of aspirin (900–1200 mg). Some patients prefer a non-steroidal anti-inflammatory drug (NSAID) or paracetamol 1000 mg. Fixed drug combinations of an antiemetic with aspirin or paracetamol are available but expensive. Domperidone has fewer side effects than other antiemetics, and is available over the counter. Rectal antiemetics or NSAIDs such as diclofenac (intramuscular injection can be helpful) are worth considering. Opiates should not be used because they worsen gastrointestinal symptoms and have abuse potential, especially in the genesis of MOH.

## Triptans

The introduction of triptans in the 1990s has revolutionized the treatment of migraine. Five triptans are currently licensed in the UK, with one or two more expected shortly. Only the licensed triptans will be discussed here. Triptans are relatively expensive; they are, on average, slightly more effective than simple analgesia with an antiemetic, when judged by number needed to treat (NNT) (Bandolier, 1999). This average response conceals substantial inter- and intra-patient variation. Some people respond well to triptans and poorly to other agents. There may be little to choose between the different triptans, which are listed in *Table 4.4*.

**Table 4.4: Triptan costs**

|  |  | Cost per tablet | NNT* | Cost per pain-free patient |
|---|---|---|---|---|
| Sumatriptan | 50 mg | £4.00 | 4.0 | £15.92 |
|  | 100 mg | £8.00 | 4.3 | £34.07 |
| Naratriptan | 2.5 mg | £4.00 | 9.2 | £36.75 |
| Zolmitriptan | 2.5 mg | £4.00 | 5.9 | £19.49 |
|  | 5 mg | £8.00 | 3.3 | £26.25 |
| Rizatriptan | 10 mg | £4.46 | 3.1 | £13.85 |
| Almotriptan | 12.5 mg | £3.25 | 4.6 | £15.00 |

*NNT=Number needed to treat, to achieve one pain-free patient 2 hours post-dose. From Belsey (2000, 2001)

⌘ Sumatriptan (Imigran, GlaxoSmithKline, Brentford) was the first to market. The tablets are the market leader in the UK, so have the advantage of familiarity. Sumatriptan is the only injectable triptan, offering the most rapid, effective and expensive therapy; its nasal spray is relatively rarely used.

⌘ Naratriptan (Naramig, GlaxoSmithKline, Brentford) is the least potent, but it has few side effects.

⌘ Zolmitriptan (Zomig, Astra Zeneca, Luton) has potentially the lowest NNT at its top dose of 5 mg.

⌘ Rizatriptan (Maxalt, Merck Sharp and Dohme, Hoddesdon) has the lowest mean NNT and the lowest cost per effectively-treated migraine (Belsey, 2000).

⌘ Almotriptan (Almogran, Lundbeck, Milton Keynes) is substantially cheaper than the other triptans, with efficacy and tolerability similar to sumatriptan (Spierings et al, 2001).

Mouth-dispersible preparations, such as Maxalt melt and Zomig rapimelt, have no proven advantage over tablets: they are not absorbed through the buccal mucosa. This formulation may be intuitively patient-friendly, without cost disadvantage.

Triptans are relatively safe drugs; concerns about cardiac toxicity have only rarely been realized in clinical practice. However, triptans should never be used in those with, or at risk of, cardiac ischaemia.

The main problems with triptans are cost, and the tendency for a minority of users (perhaps as many as 10%) to overuse them. There is certainly no place for daily triptan use, although such users are not uncommon in secondary and tertiary headache practice. The management is the same as for any other MOH: cure follows drug withdrawal, and is not facilitated by further prescriptions.

## Ergots

Ergot preparations may still have a place in the acute management of migraine, although ergot users in headache clinics almost invariably have ergot dependency, yet another type of MOH.

## Recurrence

Recurrence of migraine after initial response affects one-third of patients with migraine. Recurrence is complex and poorly understood: at the simplest level, an ineffective treatment has zero recurrence. Some authorities recommend the combination of a triptan with a NSAID to reduce recurrence risk, although this is not evidence based.

## Step care vs stratified care

Step care means starting with simple analgesia, perhaps with an antiemetic, and escalating in one or more steps toward triptans. With stratified care, low-impact migraine is treated with simple analgesia and an antiemetic, but high-impact migraine is treated first with a triptan. Stratified care results in significantly better clinical outcomes than step care, according to Lipton et al (2000), but at a higher price. This comparison assumes that the two strategies are equivalent. It is arguable that the analgesic/antiemetic approach is appropriate to use early in a migraine attack, perhaps before pain is significant, for example during aura or prodrome. Triptan licensing studies have treated migraine pain of at least moderate severity; triptans are ineffective if given before the onset of headache.

# Prevention of migraine

### Lifestyle management

Adjustment of lifestyle may be helpful, although evidence is largely anecdotal. Regularity of biorhythms is the key. Avoidance of relative hypoglycaemia with a regular, fibre-containing diet is probably the most helpful strategy. Dietary exclusion is rarely helpful and should be abandoned if ineffective. Change in sleeping times at weekends and irregular shift work may usefully be avoided; also abrupt let-down from stress. International travel is a common migraine trigger.

### Alternative therapies

Alternative therapies are often acceptable to patients, although are rarely evidence based. Feverfew, magnesium and vitamin B2 mega-doses may be effective (Silberstein, 2000), with several months latency to benefit. Manipulative treatments are ineffective unless there is associated muscle pain. Homeopathy is ineffective, according to Whitmarsh et al (1997). Acupuncture probably has only an acute analgesic effect.

### Prescribed drugs

The prevention of migraine with daily drug treatment should be considered only after acute treatment has been optimized, medication overuse abolished, lifestyle modification tried and a migraine diary recorded for 1–3 months. Most agents offer partial benefit only, which may take 1–5 months to achieve; *Table 4.5* lists those most commonly used.

**Table 4.5: Prophylactic drug treatments for migraine**

| | Start dose | Maximum dose | Side effects, comments | Alternative agents |
|---|---|---|---|---|
| Amitriptyline | 5–10 mg | 200 mg | Sedation and dry mouth | Consider other tricyclics or SSRIs |
| Propranolol | 20 mg | 320 mg | Cold limbs, nightmares | Atenolol may be better tolerated |
| Valproate | 500 mg | 1500 mg | Weight gain, teratogenicity | Consider gabapentin, topiramate |
| Methysergide | 1 mg | 8 mg | Limb pain, visceral fibrosis, 6 months treatment, 1 month break | |
| Pizotifen | 0.5 mg | 3 mg | Weight gain, sedation, low efficacy | |

NB. Many of these drugs are unlicensed in this indication. SSRI = selective serotonin-reuptake inhibitor

Patients must be informed that occurrence of migraine after starting prophylaxis does not mean treatment failure. Comorbid disease, such as depression or insomnia, may suggest amitriptyline as the initial choice; hypertension indicates a beta-blocker. It is unusual to offer prophylaxis for less than two attacks a month. Treatment should be titrated first for tolerability then for efficacy. After 6 months of effective treatment, phased withdrawal should be considered.

## Hormones and migraine

This has been comprehensively reviewed by MacGregor (2000). Migraine is more common in women, the gender difference beginning at puberty. Menstruation is a migraine trigger in 10% of women with migraine. This is often overestimated by the patient: true menstrual migraine can be diagnosed only after examining a few months of headache and menstrual diary. The oestrogen-containing contraceptive pill (OCP) may improve or less commonly exacerbate migraine, which may be troublesome in the pill-free week. Tri-cycling the OCP (continuous use for three packs) and transdermal oestrogen can help.

Migraine, especially migraine with aura, is probably an independent risk factor for stroke. However, confidence intervals of case-control studies are wide, making risk assessment difficult. This leads many authorities to question the wisdom of OCPs for women with migraine. The risk is probably low in migraine without aura.

Migraine with aura is a relative contraindication to the OCP. Intrauterine devices and progesterone-only contraceptives affect neither migraine nor stroke risk, so are preferable to OCPs for women with migraine without aura or migraine with aura.

Migraine typically improves during the second and third trimesters of pregnancy, although can be troublesome in the puerperium.

The climacteric and menopause are associated with migraine worsening, as often as with improvement. Transdermal, not oral, hormone replacement therapy is often helpful.

# References

Bandolier (1999) Making sense of migraine. Bandolier 59–2 (http://www.jr2.ox.ac.uk/bandolier/band59/b59-2.html)

Belsey J (2000) The clinical and financial impact of oral triptans in the management of migraine in the UK: a systematic review. *J Med Econ* **3**: 35–47

Belsey J (2001) Clinical efficacy and cost effectiveness of oral triptans: an updated meta-analysis incorporating data for almotriptan. Presented at the 10th Congress of the International Headache Society, New York, June 29–July 2

Elrington G (1997) 1000 headaches: how many brain scans? *Cephalalgia* **17**(3): 317

Goadsby PJ (2001) Migraine, aura and cortical spreading depression: why are we still talking about it? *Ann Neurol* **49**(2): 4–6

International Headache Society (1988) Headache classification committee of the International Headache Society. Classification and diagnostic criteria for headache disorders, cranial neuralgias and facial pain. *Cephalalgia* **8**(suppl): 7

Lipton RB, Stewart WF, Stone AM, Láinez MJA, Sawyer JPC (2000) Stratified care *vs* step care strategies for migraine. *JAMA* **284**: 2599–605

MacGregor AE (2000) Gynaecological aspects of migraine. *Rev Contemp Pharmacother* **11**: 75–90

Rasmussen BK, Stewart WF (2000) Epidemiology of migraine. In: Olesen J, Tfelt-Hansen P, Welch KMA, eds. *The Headaches*. 2nd edn. Lippincott Williams & Wilkins, Philadelphia: 227–33

Silberstein SD (2000) Practice parameter: evidence-based guidelines for migraine headache (an evidence-based review). *Neurology* **55**: 754–62

Spierings ELH, Gomez-Mancilla B, Grosz DE (2001) Oral almotriptan *vs* oral sumatriptan. A double-blind, randomized, parallel-group, optimum-dose comparison. *Arch Neurol* **58**: 944–50

Steiner TJ, MacGregor EA, Davies PTG (2001) Guidelines for all doctors in the management of migraine and tension-type headache. Available at: http://www.bash.org.uk. Accessed 8 September 2001

Whitmarsh TE, Coleston-Shields DM, Steiner TJ (1997) Double-blind randomized placebo-controlled study of homoeopathic prophylaxis of migraine. *Cephalalgia* **17**: 600–4

# Chapter 5

# Medical management of facial pain

*HC Romer*

This chapter describes some of the means used to manage facial pain once serious pathology or any treatable cause has been excluded. It includes pharmacological, physical and psychological therapies.

Some facial pain can be managed by surgical or pharmacological treatment of the cause. However, signs of serious conditions, such as cranial tumours, must be excluded before the medical management of the pain itself starts.

## Physiology of pain

The physiology described below covers facial pain originating from the neck. If one considers the brainstem to be analogous to the dorsal horn, the same explanation can be used for pain in the distribution of cranial nerves, although the physiology in these cases is more complex and less well understood.

### Ascending pathways

A$\delta$- and C-nerve fibres transmit pain from the periphery to the spinal cord. They are the smallest fibres in the myelinated and unmyelinated groups. The myelinated A$\delta$ fibres receive input from up to 20 mechanoreceptors per fibre and transmit the signal relatively fast (6–30 m/sec). They adapt rapidly to a constant stimulation, so the signal fades quickly. Conversely, each C fibre has one bare nerve ending acting as a polymodal nociceptor. Pain signals in C fibres travel at <2 m/sec to the spinal cord, and adaptation to a constant pain is slow.

Pain fibres terminate in Rexed's laminae in the dorsal root horn of the spinal cord. A series of interneurones between lamina 2 (the substantia gelatinosa) and lamina 5 allow alteration of the signal before it reaches the spinal tracts. Most pain fibres decussate to ascend in the contralateral spinothalamic tract. Connections exist with the thalamus, reticular formation, frontal lobe, hypothalamus, limbic system and sensory cortex (*Figure 5.1*).

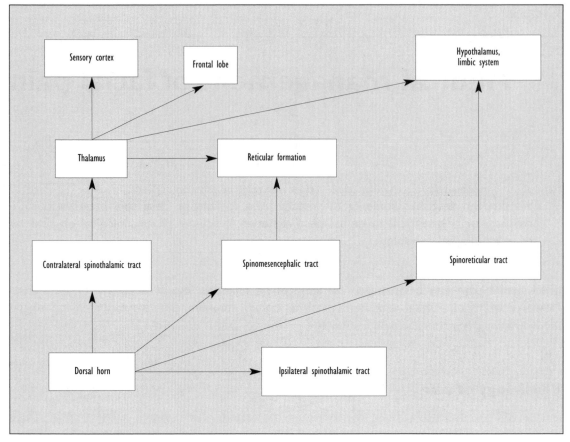

Figure 5.1: Ascending pain pathways.

### Modulation of the pain pathway and descending pathways

Researchers continue to find more pathways and neurotransmitters involved in the modulation of the ascending pain signal. Of clinical significance here are the descending tracts that decrease ascending pain signals. These are tracts relying on serotonin (5HT) and noradrenaline as their neurotransmitters.

The descending tracts are thought to interact with the ascending pain pathway at the level of the dorsal root horn. It is also at this level that the modulations explained by Melzack and Wall's gate control theory of pain occur. Sensory input from the periphery, carried by Aβ fibres, can modulate and sometimes block the pain signal travelling through the network of interneurones ('close the gate') (*Figure 5.2*). Activation of N-methyl-D-aspartate (NMDA) receptors in this region leads to 'wind up' with recruitment of more interneurones and amplification of the pain signal.

More peripheral modulation of the pain pathway tends to increase pain. Antidromic flow in C fibres and efferent sympathetic flow cause release of substance P and noradrenaline respectively. Both of these, together with local inflammatory mediators such as bradykinin and prostaglandins, sensitize peripheral receptors.

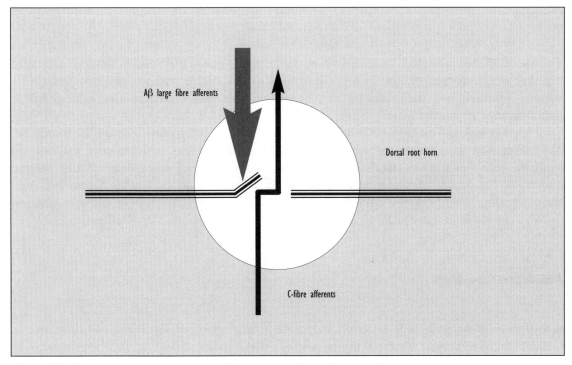

*Figure 5.2: Diagrammatic representation of the gate control theory of pain.*

## Pharmacological management of chronic pain

The World Health Organization's analgesic ladder for mild, moderate and severe pain in cancer can be used in chronic pain. Most patients will already have discarded simple analgesics. However, these are worth reviewing to check that they have been tried and also to ensure that non-steroidal anti-inflammatory drugs (NSAIDs) have not been overused, which can lead to medication misuse chronic daily headache.

### NSAIDs

NSAIDs act in the periphery by decreasing inflammatory mediators and are also thought to act centrally via receptors in the spinal cord. The cyclo-oxygenase-2 (Cox-2) inhibitors are designed to interact minimally with the 'housekeeping' Cox-1 prostaglandin receptor. They aim to have fewer gastric side effects but may increase the incidence of cardiovascular events.

Indomethacin is especially worth mentioning as it is particularly effective in the short-lived but frequent chronic paroxysmal headache (Goadsby, 1999).

## Opiates

The use of opiates in chronic facial pain is controversial. Against their use are fears of addiction together with long-term failure as a result of habituation, ineffectiveness and intolerable side effects. Research into their success in neuropathic pain has mixed results, but a trial of treatment may be worthwhile.

The oral opiates include codeine, dihydrocodeine and tramadol, as well as morphine, oxycodone and methadone for severe pain. Slow-release forms and fentanyl patches are available once the dose has stabilized. In order to avoid increasing doses, drug rotation may be employed. The patient alternates between two or three different drugs over the course of a year, thereby taking 'drug holidays' from each substance. The risk of addiction or abuse is between 0–24%, but lower in those with no previous psychiatric or abuse history (Dellemijn, 1999).

## Antidepressant drugs

Antidepressant drugs include amitriptyline, nortriptyline, doxepin, dothiepin and imipramine. Gabapentin, a structural γ-aminobutyric acid (GABA) analogue, works in a similar way to traditional antidepressants. Nortriptyline and gabapentin have fewer side effects than amitriptyline (Beydoun, 1999; Kanazi et al, 2000), and it has been suggested that they should be used first out of this group. Pregabalin may be used in place of gabapentin. Both are classed as anticonvulsant drugs.

Prescribed in lower doses than in depression, the antidepressants block the reuptake of biogenic amines, serotonin and noradrenaline in the brainstem, thereby increasing the effect of the descending modulatory spinal tracts. They also potentiate endogenous and exogenous opioids. They do not, at the dosage used in pain management, act as antidepressants, and this may need to be explained to the patient.

Antidepressants are particularly useful in pains of a burning nature, tension (Cerbo et al, 1998) and cluster headaches, as well as in allodynia. They should be started at a low dose and increased gradually as benefits and side-effects dictate. Unwanted effects include thirst, constipation and dysphoria. Taken at night, drowsiness is an advantage. Other benefits may take 2–3 weeks to be noticeable.

## Selective serotonin-reuptake inhibitors

This newer class of antidepressants includes fluoxetine, paroxetine and citalopram. They are used in the same way as older antidepressants but avoid the noradrenergic side effects of these drugs.

Sumatriptan is a cranioselective serotonin agonist of particular use in migraine. It has not shown clinical benefit in atypical facial pain.

### Ion channel blockers

### Anticonvulsant drugs

Carbamazepine, clonazepam, phenytoin and sodium valproate block sodium channels in active nerves, thereby decreasing the spontaneous impulses that can occur in damaged C-fibres, which patients describe as 'stabbing' or 'sharp' pain (such as in trigeminal neuralgia) or an unpleasant 'pins and needles' sensation. Carbamazepine is the drug of first choice for the treatment of trigeminal neuralgia.

### Others

Lignocaine infusions can relieve neuropathic pain, but as they are unavailable orally they are not clinically useful in chronic pain. Topical lignocaine has been successful in treating postherpetic neuralgia (Comer and Lamb, 2000).

Oral mexiletine has had mixed results.

Lamotrigine stabilizes a subtype of sodium channels and suppresses neuronal release of glutamate. It can be used alone or in combination with carbamazepine in the treatment of neuralgia (Sindrup and Jensen, 1999).

### NMDA antagonists

Ketamine is a non-competitive NMDA receptor antagonist that is thought to minimize the wind-up phenomenon. Intravenous ketamine has had good results in the treatment of neuropathic pain, and results of trials on the oral form are awaited.

Oral dextromethorphan has a lower receptor affinity and is usually unsuccessful in treating facial pain.

The synthetic opiates, methadone and tramadol, block NMDA receptors in addition to their effects on opiate receptors.

### Sedatives and antispasmodics

Diazepam can be of use in chronic orofacial muscle pain (Singer and Dionne, 1997). This may be as a result of its antispasmodic or anxiolytic effects.

Baclofen, a GABA-receptor agonist that is usually used as an antispasmodic, has been shown to be useful in the treatment of central pain neuralgias (arising after brain injury), cluster headaches (Hering-Hanit and Gadoth, 2000) and chronic daily headache from medication misuse.

## *Miscellaneous drugs*

### *Capsaicin*

The alkaloid capsaicin, applied as a cream to the hypersensitive area, causes release of substance P from sensory nerve terminals and also has effects in the spinal cord, possibly as a result of absorption or neuronal transport. Used regularly, this results in a depletion of substance P and a decrease in paraesthesia, dysaesthesia and allodynia (Lincoff et al, 1998). As the initial treatments are painful, it may be prescribed with EMLA cream for the first few days, and needs to be used regularly.

### *Oxygen and ergotamine*

Thought to cause transient cerebral vasoconstriction, oxygen can abort a cluster headache as can inhaled (nasal spray) or subcutaneous ergotamine (A Leach, personal communication, 2000).

### *Lithium carbonate*

Lithium may be used in the prophylactic treatment for chronic cluster headaches, but plasma levels must be monitored.

# Physical management of chronic pain

### *Transcutaneous electrical nerve stimulation*

Using an electric current that is passed between two electrodes attached to the skin, transcutaneous electrical nerve stimulation (TENS) stimulates Aβ fibres and therefore modulates the pain sensation at the level of the dorsal root horn. With experimentation, the settings can be adjusted so that all sensation of pain is lost while the TENS machine is used and sometimes for some hours afterwards.

Drawbacks include difficulty in attaching the electrodes and skin reactions to the electrode glue. TENS should be tried for a variety of conditions; however, it is of particular use in myofascial pain deriving from neck and strap muscles.

### Physiotherapy

Physiotherapy aims to restore normal muscle function, and it is of most benefit in myofascial pain where trigger points in the neck muscles cause radiation to distant areas (*Figure 5.3*).

Stretching, mobilization, cooling sprays or ice are used with local anaesthetic

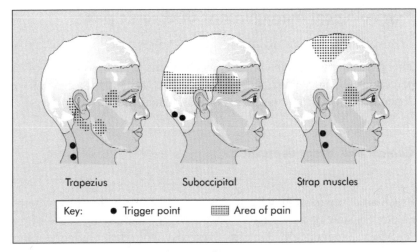

*Figure 5.3: Trigger points and pain radiation.*

injections and acupuncture. Where bruxism contributes to continued muscle malfunction, dental splints may be use.

### Acupuncture

Acupuncture is used in its traditional form and in trigger point treatment. It has been successfully used in postherpetic neuralgia and atypical facial pain. Studies have shown that some of the benefits gained from acupuncture may be the result of patient motivation and placebo effect (McMillan et al, 1997).

### Nerve blockade

Bupivacaine can be used to block the greater occipital and supraorbital nerves and cervical facet joints to treat cervicogenic headaches.

In order to abort a cluster headache, patients can be taught to perform a sphenopalatine block by positioning two cotton buds soaked in local anaesthetic inside the nose.

### Botulinum toxin

Botulinum injection into the masseter muscle can relieve spasm in temporomandibular dysfunction, but should be carried out by someone experienced in this technique.

# Psychological management of chronic pain

The psychological state, coping mechanisms and personality of the patient will affect the perception of pain. Pain, in turn, will affect the patient's mental wellbeing. Ignoring this co-dependence will limit the success of pain management.

## Clinical and latent depression

Psychiatric treatment may be necessary for the few patients for whom severe clinical depression, an anxiety state or a personality disorder is the underlying cause of pain.

Most patients will benefit from psychological support, ranging from a sympathetic consultation with a doctor who acknowledges their pain to active psychotherapy (Haythornthwaite and Benrud-Larson, 2000).

## Cognitive–behavioural therapy

Chronic pain has been compared with a phobia, where the patient learns that a particular activity or movement causes pain. Over time, this can build up to the point where even thinking of the activity brings on the pain. Cognitive–behavioural therapy, together with biofeedback, seeks to support patients while they change their behaviour, learn to pace themselves and complete tasks by alternate means.

## Education

A deeper understanding of the mechanism of pain and the idea that 'hurt' does not automatically equal 'harm' can benefit most patients. Exploration of the emotional and social impact of pain and an insight into pain behaviour increase patients' understanding of the condition and decrease fear and pain.

## Relaxation and hypnosis

Relaxation can be used as prophylactic pain management in stress avoidance and can be combined with physical and psychological therapies. Hypnosis can be of help in pain that is resistant to other treatments (Simon and Lewis, 2000).

## Other alternative therapies

Other alternative therapies include homeopathy, Reike, aromatherapy and reflexology. The success of each therapy is individual and may owe much to patient motivation and the effect of a compassionate, interested practitioner. Some patients receive remarkable benefit from these other alternative therapies, but the scientific basis of these therapies has yet to be elucidated.

Osteopaths and chiropractors use treatments similar to manipulative physiotherapy.

## Conclusion

Serious, treatable causes of pain must be excluded. Pain treatment relies on the integration of pharmacological, physical and psychological support. Pain management programmes seek to provide this and increase patients' self-reliance so that they can retake control of their management and future.

## References

Beydoun A (1999) Postherpetic neuralgia: role of gabapentin and other treatment modalities. *Epilepsia* **40(6)**: S51–6

Cerbo R, Barbanti P, Fabbrini G, Pascali MP, Catarci T (1998) Amitriptyline is effective in chronic but not in episodic tension-type headache: pathogenetic implications. *Headache* **38(6)**: 453–7

Comer AM, Lamb HM (2000) Lidocaine patch 5%. *Drugs* **59(2)**: 245–9

Dellemijn P (1999) Are opioids effective in relieving neuropathic pain? *Pain* **80(3)**: 453–62

Goadsby PJ (1999) Short-lasting primary headaches: focus on trigeminal automatic cephalgias and indomethacin-sensitive headaches. *Curr Opin Neurol* **12(3)**: 273–7

Haythornthwaite JA, Benrud-Larson LM (2000) Psychological aspects of neuropathic pain. *Clin J Pain* **16(2 Suppl)**: S101–5

Hering-Hanit R, Gadoth N (2000) Baclofen in cluster headache. *Headache* **40(1)**: 48–51

Kanazi GE, Johnson RW, Dworkin RH (2000) Treatment of postherpetic neuralgia: an update. *Drugs* **59(5)**: 1113–26

Lincoff NS, Rath PP, Hirano M (1998) The treatment of periocular and facial pain with topical capsaicin. *J Neuro-Ophthalmol* **18(1)**: 17–20

McMillan AS, Nolan A, Kelly PJ (1997) The efficacy of dry needling and procaine in the treatment of myofascial pain in the jaw muscles. *J Orofacial Pain* **11(4)**: 307–14

Simon EP, Lewis DM (2000) Medical hypnosis for temporomandibular disorders: treatment efficacy and medical utilization outcome. *Oral Surg Oral Med Oral Pathol Oral Radiol Endod* **90(1)**: 54–63

Sindrup SH, Jensen TS (1999) Efficacy of pharmacological treatments of neuropathic pain: an update and effect related to mechanism of drug action. *Pain* **83**: 389–400

Singer E, Dionne R (1997) A controlled evaluation of ibuprofen and diazepam for chronic orofacial muscle pain. *J Orofacial Pain* **11(2)**: 139–46

Chapter 6

# Managing side effects of radiotherapy in head and neck cancer

*RL Mendes, CM Nutting, KJ Harrington*

Curative radiotherapy for head and neck cancer causes significant side effects. In addition to their considerable impact on the patient's quality of life, these effects can prejudice treatment outcome. This chapter looks at the management of the adverse effects of radiotherapy for head and neck cancer.

Radiotherapy frequently cures head and neck cancer, but at the expense of significant side effects caused by radiation-induced damage to normal tissues. These radiation reactions may be classified as early and late:

- Early reactions occur during and/or shortly after treatment and may persist for up to 3 months
- Late reactions occur months to years after the treatment.

However, this classification is not clear-cut. Certain predictable reactions (e.g. dry mouth) occur acutely and persist as a permanent late effect. Alternatively, an exaggerated acute reaction may fail to resolve and persist as a chronic consequential effect (Denham et al, 1999). The common acute and late effects of radiotherapy for head and neck cancer are listed in *Table 6.1*.

The importance of acute reactions is that they have a significant impact on the patient's quality of life (QoL) and may delay, or even prevent, delivery of a full curative radiation dose. Such changes to the normal time-course of radiation dose delivery can result in significant reductions in the likelihood of cure. In contrast, late reactions only evolve after treatment is completed, have a chronic, debilitating effect on the patient's QoL and may, on occasions, be life threatening. Therefore, in an attempt to reduce radiotherapy-induced side effects, strenuous efforts are made to limit the amount of normal tissue that is irradiated. However, in order to treat the tumour it is frequently necessary to risk a degree of normal tissue damage. Therefore, a certain level of risk for some potential complications must be accepted and discussed with the patient.

This chapter gives an understanding of the biological principles that govern the pathogenesis and management of acute and late toxicity. It looks at the common acute and late reactions seen in the clinical setting and discusses their management in the context of a multidisciplinary team.

## Table 6.1: Early and late side effects of radiotherapy

| | |
|---|---|
| **Early** | Mucositis |
| | Desquamation |
| | Xerostomia |
| | Alopecia |
| | Loss of taste |
| | Lhermitte's phenomenon |
| **Late** | Xerostomia |
| | Osteoradionecrosis |
| | Fibrosis |
| | Soft tissue necrosis |
| | Neurological damage |
| | Second malignancy |

## Radiotherapy-induced tissue damage

The target of radiation in both cancerous and normal cells is DNA. Damage occurs either through a direct or an indirect effect.

The direct effect is rare and is caused by a radiation beam depositing its energy directly in a DNA molecule. More commonly, the indirect effect results from a radiation beam depositing its energy in a water molecule to form free radicals (highly reactive molecules that can damage DNA). This DNA damage, if sufficiently severe, can trigger cell death.

Actively dividing cells (e.g. skin, mucosa, hair follicles) are most sensitive to radiotherapy, and their death causes the acute reaction. In contrast, non-dividing cells (e.g. connective tissue, bone) do not manifest their accumulated DNA damage unless called upon to divide, dying a so-called 'mitotic death' at a later date. Cells contain scavenger molecules (e.g. glutathione) that can mop up free radicals and limit DNA damage.

In addition, both normal and cancer cells can repair DNA damage, although it is hoped that malignant cells do this less effectively. By dividing a course of radiotherapy into 30–35 separate fractions over 6–7 weeks, this differential in the ability to repair DNA damage is magnified, with the result that the tumour can be cured without completely destroying the surrounding normal tissues.

# Factors affecting radiation reactions

The degree of radiation reaction can be influenced by treatment- and patient-related factors.

## *Treatment factors*

Radiotherapy-induced toxicity is directly proportional to the total radiation dose delivered and the volume of tissue that is irradiated. In addition, the dose delivered per treatment fraction is important, especially for late reactions. It is this fact that underlies the use of protracted courses of small fractions of radiation over many weeks.

Different types of radiation deposit their dose at different depths within tissue. Low-energy (superficial) X-rays (50–200 KeV) and electrons deposit a higher proportion of their dose at the skin surface compared with high-energy X-rays and γ-rays (1–10 MV). Therefore, skin toxicity is reduced when high-energy X-rays and γ-rays are used.

Patients with advanced head and neck cancer often receive concurrent chemotherapy and radiotherapy. This approach certainly increases acute reactions and may accentuate late reactions.

## *Patient factors*

Some rare genetic disorders relating to the repair of DNA damage cause increased radiation reactions (*Table 6.2*). Acquired disorders, which can affect patients with head and neck cancer, include conditions that affect tissue repair (e.g. poor nutritional status, high alcohol intake, smoking). Reduced levels of scavenger molecules (in such conditions as human immunodeficiency virus (HIV) infection or acquired immunodeficiency syndrome (AIDS)) may also increase reactions (Costleigh et al, 1995; Formenti et al, 1995).

---

**Table 6.2: Genetic syndromes associated with increased sensitivity to radiation**

---

Ataxia telangiectasia

Gardner's syndrome

Fanconi's anaemia

Severe combined immunodeficiency syndrome

Xeroderma pigmentosum

---

# Acute side effects

## *Mucositis*

Mucositis occurs through death of stem cells in the basal layer of the non-keratinized epithelium of the upper aerodigestive tract. Because the stem cells renew the epithelium every 2 weeks or so, the acute reaction is not observed until the third week of treatment when the lack of replacement epithelial cells becomes apparent.

There are four recognized phases (*Table 6.3*) and grades (*Table 6.4*) for mucositis.

**Table 6.3: The four phases of radiation-induced mucositis**

| | |
|---|---|
| **The inflammatory phase** | Cytokine release (mainly tumour necrosis factor-$\alpha$, interleukin-1 and interleukin-6) by the epithelium and surrounding connective tissue causes tissue damage |
| **The epithelial phase** | Manifest by atrophy and ulceration as the damaged basal cell layer migrates to the surface and is exposed |
| **The ulcerative phase** | Fibrinous pseudomembranes cover areas of ulceration. There is colonization with Gram-negative organisms with endotoxin and cytokine release, causing more damage to the epithelium |
| **The healing phase** | The epithelium regenerates as the basal cell layer proliferates and the normal microflora is established |

**Table 6.4: Grading of mucositis**

| | |
|---|---|
| **Grade 0** | No change over baseline |
| **Grade 1** | Hyperaemia |
| **Grade 2** | Patchy mucositis |
| **Grade 3** | Confluent mucositis |
| **Grade 4** | Ulceration, haemorrhage, necrosis |

A representative example of a grade 3 mucositis of the soft palate is shown in *Figure 6.1.*

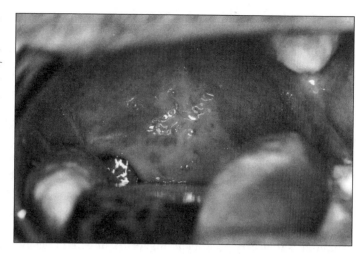

*Figure 6.1: Grade 3 radiation mucositis affecting the soft palate. This is a direct view into the oral cavity with a tongue depressor (bottom of picture) in place. Confluent mucosal reaction can be seen over the soft palate with evidence of a yellow/white pseudomembrane and increased vascularity (small dilated blood vessels are seen at the margin of the reaction). The tongue, which is seen at the bottom of the picture bulging either side of the tongue depressor, has significant overlying slough.*

## Management of mucositis

There are no effective means of preventing the occurrence of radiotherapy-induced mucositis (Symonds, 1998). Hence, care is taken during the planning process to ensure maximal shielding of mucosa from radiation beams, without compromising tumour coverage. Once present there is no established treatment to accelerate the resolution of mucositis, although several measures are recommended to alleviate symptoms.

The mainstay of therapy is the use of oral analgesics, which are prescribed according to the World Health Organization analgesic ladder (*Figure 6.2*). Although frequently prescribed, there is no convincing support for the use of mouthwashes (Feber, 1996). Normal saline and sodium bicarbonate are used, especially if there is extensive slough. Mouthwashes containing alcohol are avoided as they may increase local inflammation and cause pain. Likewise, the patient is advised to avoid alcohol and smoking during treatment.

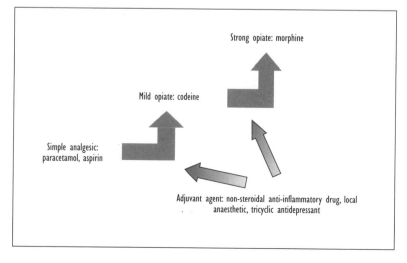

Strong opiate: morphine

Mild opiate: codeine

Simple analgesic: paracetamol, aspirin

Adjuvant agent: non-steroidal anti-inflammatory drug, local anaesthetic, tricyclic antidepressant

*Figure 6.2. Analgesia for mucositis: the World Health Organization analgesic ladder.*

## Cytoprotectants

*Sucralfate.* This agent forms ionic bonds with proteins within an ulcer and acts as a protective barrier. It may also aid healing by increasing local prostaglandin $E_2$ release (Ferraro and Mattern, 1984).

*Topical non-steroidal anti-inflammatory drugs.* A large, double-blind, placebo-controlled trial of benzydamine reported decreased pain scores for patients on the active compound (Epstein and Stevenson-Moore, 1986). Indomethacin given on the first day of treatment has also been shown to decrease the severity and onset of mucositis (Pillsbury et al, 1986).

*Steroids.* The role of corticosteroid mouthwashes is unclear. A few non-randomized trials suggest they may be useful (Abdelaal et al, 1989; Rothwell and Spektor, 1990), but the risk of oral candidiasis that may accentuate mucositis must be considered.

*Growth factors.* Granulocyte-macrophage colony-stimulating factor (GM-CSF) is an endogenous 14 KDa protein that acts on connective tissue, triggering release of fibroblast growth factor and interleukin-1, which stimulate the basal layer to proliferate. A small, randomized trial of this agent administered subcutaneously in patients with laryngeal cancer demonstrated that it reduced mucositis of the upper aerodigestive tract (J McAleese, personal communication, 2002). An ongoing Radiation Therapy Oncology Group trial is addressing similar issues. Topical GM-CSF mouthwash has no role to play (Sprinzl et al, 2001).

*Antimicrobials.* Patients undergoing treatment may develop oropharyngeal candidal infections because of poor oral hygiene and reduced mucosal defence mechanisms. Candida is treated with nystatin mouthwash, or oral fluconazole in cases of persistent infection. At present, there is no established prophylactic role for antifungal and antibacterial antimicrobials. Polymyxin E and tobramycin are active against Gram-negative organisms that frequently colonize and promote mucositis by endotoxin release. There is evidence that selective depletion of Gram-negative organisms by antibiotic lozenges can decrease mucositis (Spijkervet et al, 1991).

*Silver nitrate.* This agent stimulates cell division in normal mucosa. There are conflicting data on its role in managing mucositis (Maciejewski et al, 1991; Dorr et al, 1995).

*Modulators of oxidative stress.* Gluthathione and amifostine work by mopping up free radicals. Therefore, they may reduce the acute radiation reaction. There are limited data relating to their effect in preventing mucositis.

## Xerostomia

The major salivary glands produce up to 90% of saliva. The position and size of the parotid gland means that it is frequently included in the radiation treatment field for head and neck cancer. The serous acini (which produce watery saliva) are more sensitive to the effects of radiotherapy than the mucous acini, resulting in the production of thick, tenacious saliva. The decrease in the quantity and quality of saliva may lead to a change in oral flora and accelerated dental caries.

The free-radical scavenger amifostine accumulates preferentially in salivary tissue. It has been shown to reduce acute and chronic xerostomia without adversely affecting the anti-tumour effects of radiotherapy. Amifostine is expensive and may cause nausea, vomiting, hypotension and rarely allergic reactions (Schuchter, 1996). More recently, there has been significant progress in the use of intensity-modulated radiotherapy as a means of sparing the parotid gland from receiving high radiation doses in patients with head and neck cancer. Otherwise, the management of xerostomia is palliative. Patients should sip water regularly or use artificial saliva. In severe cases, oral pilocarpine can improve symptoms (LeVeque et al, 1993), although unpleasant cholinergic side effects are often limiting.

## Altered sense of taste

Dysgeusia occurs because of radiotherapy-induced damage to the circumvallate and the fungiform papillae of the tongue. The taste buds mediating bitter or sour taste are affected more than those for sweet or salty taste. The extent of sensory disturbance is directly related to the volume of the tongue that is irradiated (Fernando et al, 1995). Complete or partial recovery is usual, but can be slow and may take months to resolve. This symptom can be distressing to the patient and is rather poorly understood.

## Maintaining nutrition

Mucositis, xerostomia and dysgeusia all contribute to a decrease in oral intake. Many patients with head and neck cancer have a pre-existing poor nutritional state. Management of this problem involves a multidisciplinary team including the oncologist, dietician, pain control team and gastroenterologist. In some circumstances, a nasogastric or percutaneous endoscopic gastrostomy tube is required to maintain nutrition while the acute reactions settle.

## Acute skin reactions

Attempts are usually made to limit the acute radiation effects in the skin by using high-energy X-rays or γ-rays that deposit their maximal dose 1–2 cm below the skin surface (the so-called skin-sparing or build-up effect). However, certain sites (e.g. back of pinna, skin over laryngeal promontory) are particularly prone to acute skin reactions because of loss of a normal skin-sparing effect. In addition, in order to immobilize patients and ensure day-to-day reproducibility during radiotherapy, a personalized perspex shell is used, which has the effect of negating the skin-sparing effect and increasing the dose that is delivered to the skin. The perspex shell can be cut out in areas that do not compromise the tumour dose to prevent skin soreness. Other types of radiation, such as electrons, are often used and deposit a higher percentage of their dose at the skin surface. Skin reactions can be graded as in *Table 6.5,* and are managed as shown in *Table 6.6.*

## Table 6.5: Grading of skin reactions

| | |
|---|---|
| **Grade 0** | No reaction |
| **Grade I** | Faint erythema |
| **Grade II** | Moderate/brisk erythema, dry desquamation |
| **Grade III** | Moist desquamation |
| **Grade IV** | Skin necrosis, full thickness ulceration |

## Table 6.6: Management of acute skin reactions

| | |
|---|---|
| **Avoid irritants** | Strong soaps, sunlight |
| **Avoid local trauma** | Non-abrasive towels, loose-fitting clothing |
| **Dry desquamation** | Keep skin moisturized with aqueous cream |
| | 1% Hydrocortisone cream |
| **Moist desquamation** | Proflavine |
| | Geliperm dressings (Geislich Sons Ltd, Chester, UK) |
| | Treat secondary infections |

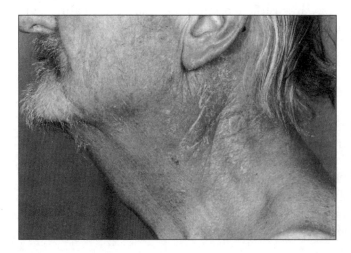

Typical dry and moist desquamation reactions are depicted in *Figures 6.3* and *6.4,* respectively.

*Figure 6.3: Radiation-induced skin reaction. There is erythema (grade 1) affecting the skin from the level of the mandible to the mid-neck below the thyroid promontory. In addition, there are areas of dry scaling of the skin (dry desquamation — grade 2), especially affecting the area of skin below the ear lobe.*

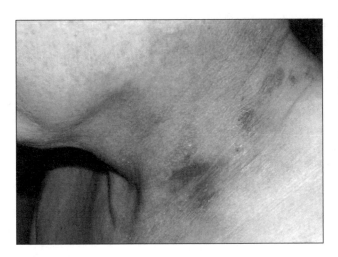

*Figure 6.4: A patient with moist desquamation (grade 3) in the skin of the left side of the neck. Areas of superficial ulceration are seen, which tend to weep and can become secondarily infected.*

### Alopecia

Alopecia occurs because the stem cells in the hair follicles are sensitive to radiotherapy. The pattern is confined within the boundaries of the radiation fields, but beam exit sites can also be affected. In treatment of head and neck cancer, alopecia is usually transient; but it may be permanent in areas of high dose.

### Neurological side effects

Lhermitte's phenomenon is manifest by tingling in the arms and legs, especially when the neck is flexed. It is thought to be caused by transient radiotherapy-induced demyelination, and is self-limiting.

## Late side effects

### Osteoradionecrosis

Osteoradionecrosis occurs when bone cells are called upon to divide in response to trauma (e.g. dental extraction) weeks, months or even years after radiotherapy. The cells then express their DNA damage and fail to heal the wound, resulting in bone necrosis. Osteoradionecrosis predominantly affects the mandible and maxilla (being 24 times commoner in the former). The pathogenesis is one of hypocellularity, hypoxia and hypovascularity. The incidence is related to the total dose received and the dose per fraction.

### Prevention and management of osteoradionecrosis

In order to reduce the risk of osteoradionecrosis, patients are advised to have all preventive and restorative dental work carried out before radiotherapy. Good oral hygiene needs to be maintained during and after completion of radiotherapy. If dental work needs to be carried out, it must be performed by an experienced dental surgeon. Once present, osteoradionecrosis poses a difficult management problem. In most cases, healing will eventually take place with conservative measures (good hygiene, adequate nutrition and prolonged courses of antibiotics), although this can be extremely slow. Debridement of bony sequestra is sometimes required. In these situations, there may be a role for adjuvant hyperbaric oxygen.

### Soft tissue fibrosis and necrosis

Fibrosis of soft tissue is a common problem after radiotherapy for head and neck cancer. The tissue becomes progressively thicker and woody-hard, limiting movement and causing disfigurement. There may be a role for the use of oxypentifylline, which has been used to treat fibrosis at other sites. Necrosis manifests as an ulcer that fails to heal. It is sometimes difficult to distinguish clinically from recurrent disease, and biopsies may be necessary. The management is conservative, keeping the area clean to prevent secondary infection.

### Second malignancy

As well as treating cancer, radiation may cause second malignancies. The most common types of second malignancies are skin cancers and sarcomas. The increased risk is estimated at approximately 1% per decade.

### Late radiation-induced neuropathy

The tolerance of peripheral nerves for radiotherapy is higher than for the central nervous system, and acute side effects are not commonly seen. Late-onset neuropathies are caused by a combination of demyelination, fibrosis and vascular degeneration.

## Conclusions

Radiotherapy is an important curative treatment for head and neck cancers, but comes at the price of significant early and late side effects. Careful management of these side effects improves the tolerability of treatment. Multidisciplinary approaches to treating these side effects gives the best chance of prompt resolution of acute effects and reduction in the risk of late effects.

# References

Abdelaal AS, Barker DS, Fergusson MM (1989) Treatment for irradiation-induced mucositis. *Lancet* **i**(8629): 97

Costleigh BJ, Miyamoto CT, Micaily B, Brady LW (1995) Heightened sensitivity of the esophagus to radiation in a patient with AIDS. *Am J Gastroenterol* **90**(5): 812–14

Denham JW, Peters LJ, Johansen J et al (1999) Do acute mucosal reactions lead to consequential late reactions in patients with head and neck cancer? *Radiother Oncol* **52**(2): 157–64

Dorr W, Jacubek A, Kummermehr J, Herrmann T, Dolling-Jochem I, Eckelt U (1995) Effects of stimulated repopulation on oral mucositis during conventional radiotherapy. *Radiother Oncol* **37**(2): 100–7

Epstein JB, Stevenson-Moore P (1986) Benzydamine hydrochloride in prevention and management of pain in oral mucositis associated with radiation therapy. *Oral Surg Oral Med Oral Pathol* **62**(2): 145–8

Feber T (1996) Management of mucositis in oral irradiation. *Clin Oncol (R Coll Radiol)* **8**: 106–11

Fernando IN, Patel T, Billingham L, Hammond C, Hallmark S, Glaholm J, Henk JM (1995) The effect of head and neck irradiation on taste dysfunction: a prospective study. *Clin Oncol (R Coll Radiol)* **7**(3): 173–8

Ferraro JM, Mattern JQ 2nd (1984) Sucralfate suspension for stomatitis. *Drug Intell Clin Pharm* **18**(2): 153

Formenti SC, Chak L, Gill P, Buess EM, Hill CK (1995) Increased radiosensitivity of normal tissue fibroblasts in patients with acquired immunodeficiency syndrome (AIDS) and with Kaposi's sarcoma. *Int J Radiat Biol* **68**(4): 411–12

LeVeque FG, Montgomery M, Potter D et al (1993) A multicenter, randomized, double-blind, placebo-controlled, dose-titration study of oral pilocarpine for treatment of radiation-induced xerostomia in head and neck cancer patients. *J Clin Oncol* **11**(6): 1124–31

Maciejewski B, Zajusz A, Pilecki B et al (1991) Acute mucositis in the stimulated oral mucosa of patients during radiotherapy for head and neck cancer. *Radiother Oncol* **22**(1): 7–11

Pillsbury HC 3rd, Webster WP, Rosenman J (1986) Prostaglandin inhibitor and radiotherapy in advanced head and neck cancers. *Arch Otolaryngol Head Neck Surg* **112**(5): 552–3

Rothwell BR, Spektor WS (1990) Palliation of radiation-related mucositis. *Spec Care Dentist* **10**(1): 21–5

Schuchter LM (1996) Guidelines for the administration of amifostine. *Semin Oncol* **23**(4 suppl 8): 40–3

Spijkervet FK, van Saene HK, van Saene JJ, Panders AK, Vermey A Mehta DM (1991) Mucositis prevention by selective elimination of oral flora in irradiated head and neck cancer patients. *J Oral Pathol Med* **19**(10): 486–9

Sprinzl GM, Galvan O, de Vries A et al (2001) Local application of granulocyte-macrophage colony stimulating factor (GM-CSF) for the treatment of oral mucositis. *Eur J Cancer* **37**(16): 2003–9

Symonds RP (1998) Treatment-induced mucositis: an old problem with new remedies. *Br J Cancer* **77**(10): 1689–95

## Chapter 7

# Management of a lump in the neck

*Nicholas J Roland, John Fenton, Rajiv K Bhalla*

This chapter reviews the management of adults who present with a neck lump, and discusses the potential causes and relevant investigations. The review emphasizes the avoidance of open biopsy and need for early referral to the appropriate specialist.

The old surgical aphorism —

*'Consider the anatomical structures and then the pathology that can arise from these'*

— is never more appropriate than when one contemplates the causes of a lump in the neck. However, one of the most important considerations in an adult presenting with a neck lump is that the mass may represent a metastatic deposit from a primary cancer.

Although the adverse effects of incisional or excisional biopsy are well documented in the literature, its practice regrettably still continues.

## Classification

It is difficult to present an exhaustive list of the potential causes of a lump in the neck, but a simple classification is illustrated in *Table 7.1*.

### Neoplastic cervical lymphadenopathy

The incidence of neoplastic cervical lymphadenopathy increases with age, and approximately 75% of lateral neck masses in patients older than 40 years are caused by malignant tumours. In the Liverpool series (Jones et al, 1993) we found that 74% of enlarged cervical nodes had developed from head and neck primary sites, and only 11% had come from primary sites outside that region. Thorough examination of the upper aerodigestive tract (to include the oral cavity, postnasal space, pharynx and larynx) and the thyroid gland is therefore mandatory.

**Table 7.1: Causes of neck lumps**

| | |
|---|---|
| **Congenital** | Lymphangiomas |
| | Dermoids |
| | Thyroglossal cysts |
| **Developmental** | Branchial cysts |
| | Laryngoceles |
| | Pharyngeal pouches |
| **Skin and subcutaneous tissue** | Sebaceous cyst |
| | Lipoma |
| **Tumours of the parapharyngeal space** | Deep lobe parotid |
| | Chemodectoma |
| **Thyroid swellings** | Multinodular goitre |
| | Solitary thyroid nodule |
| **Salivary gland tumours** | Pleomorphic adenoma |
| | Warthin's tumour |
| **Reactive neck lymphadenopathy** | Tonsillitis |
| | Glandular fever |
| | Human immunodeficiency virus |
| **Malignant neck node** | Carcinoma metastases (unknown primary) |
| | Lymphoma |

*Primary of unknown origin*

'Primary of unknown origin' is a term applied to patients with a metastatic carcinoma in cervical lymph nodes with an occult primary. A careful search will usually reveal the primary tumour in the skin or mucosal surfaces of the head and neck, or rarely in an area below the clavicles, such as the lungs. It is important to thoroughly search for the primary tumour by all available diagnostic methods, including history, physical examination, imaging, panendoscopy and selective biopsies from high-risk sites (nasopharynx, ipsilateral tonsil excision, base of tongue and piriform fossa). In approximately 3–11% of cases, the primary tumour remains elusive, and it is these that the term 'primary of unknown origin' should be reserved. The prognosis varies from a 30–70% 5-year survival. The prognosis depends on N stage (node status) and position of the node. Supraclavicular nodes have the worst prognosis, probably because many of these represent distant metastases from non-head and neck sites (e.g. lung or stomach). Patients who have a neck dissection and radiation therapy to both sides of the neck and the mucosal surfaces have better neck and local control than those who do not have such extensive treatment. However, this does not seem to translate into prolonged survival. Chemotherapy may have a place in improving this situation.

## Dermoid cysts

Dermoid cysts are midline swellings that do not move with swallowing or tongue protrusion.

## Thyroglossal cysts

Thyroglossal cysts form along the tract of the obliterated thyroglossal duct. They move with swallowing and tongue protrusion, as they are ultimately attached on their deep aspect to the larynx. Thyroglossal cysts should not be incised and drained, as this may cause an ugly sinus that is difficult to excise *in toto* and in continuity with the deflated cyst. They should be excised with the body of the hyoid bone (Sistrunks procedure). There is a high risk of recurrence if only the cyst is excised, as a tract going behind, in front or through the hyoid bone may be left behind.

## Branchial cysts

Branchial cysts arise from elements of squamous epithelium within a lymph node. They usually present in young adults, 60% on the left and 60% in males. Most arise along the line of the deep cervical lymph nodes, the anterior border of sternomastoid, at the junction of its upper third and lower two thirds. In a patient over the age of 40 years it is mandatory to exclude a potential metastatic cystic lymph node before considering excision (Flanagan et al, 1994). Failure to recognize this is a common error.

## Lymphangiomas

Lymphangiomas can be simple (thin-walled channels), cavernous (dilated lymphatic spaces) or a cystic hygroma (cysts of varying sizes). Simple and cavernous lesions arise principally in the lips, cheek and floor of the mouth. Cystic hygromas usually arise in the lower neck. Treatment is by surgical excision. Injection of sclerosants and radiotherapy have been suggested, but are not recommended.

## Pharyngeal pouches

Pharyngeal pouches are most frequently seen in the elderly. They cause a sensation of a lump in the throat, long-standing dysphagia, regurgitation of undigested food, halitosis, weight loss and recurrent chest infections as a result of aspiration. Hoarseness is unusual, but may occur as a result of irritation of the vocal cords from repeated aspiration, or more rarely as a result of involvement of the recurrent laryngeal nerve by a carcinoma arising in the pouch. Approximately 0.5–1% of all pouches have an invasive squamous cell carcinoma in their wall. Swelling in the neck may be present and is nearly always on the left side. It may gurgle on palpation and empty on external pressure. After the diagnosis is established, patients are usually treated by endoscopic stapling. The surgeon must be prepared to open the neck and repair the pharynx if stapling is not possible or a perforation occurs.

## Laryngoceles

Laryngoceles usually occur in men with a mean age of 55 years. They arise from the laryngeal saccule, expanding internally to present in the vallecula or externally through the thyrohyoid membrane. They are occasionally associated with a ventricular carcinoma.

An intermittent neck swelling is the usual presentation, perhaps with hoarseness, cough or pain. It is usually impalpable but may become both visible and palpable on performing the Valsalva manoeuvre. It may obstruct the larynx, so the safest treatment is excision, which includes the upper half of thyroid cartilage on the side of the laryngocele so that its neck can be ligated.

## Thyroid lumps

Thyroid lumps often occur as a result of nodular goitre. A solitary thyroid nodule may represent a nodule from a multinodular goitre, an adenoma or a carcinoma. Papillary carcinoma can be multifocal. Clinical assessment will reveal a lump that is in the thyroid gland position and moves on swallowing. The patient's thyroid status (e.g. euthyroid), retrosternal extension, vocal cord mobility and the presence of any cervical nodes should all be documented.

## Salivary gland lesions

Salivary gland lesions tend to emanate from the parotid or submandibular gland. The position of the lump, intra-oral examination of the salivary duct (with bimanual palpation) and facial nerve function should all be assessed. The neck should always be examined for nodes. Eighty per cent of all salivary tumours are benign: 80% occur in the parotid; and 80% are pleomorphic adenoma. Facial paralysis and neck nodes would suggest a possible adenoid cystic carcinoma.

# Anatomy

Neck lumps should always be described first in respect of their anatomical position. The neck is conventionally divided into anatomical triangles. The anterior triangle is bounded by the midline, the body of the mandible and the sternocleidomastoid muscle; the posterior triangle by the posterior border of the sternocleidomastoid muscle, the clavicle and the anterior border of the trapezius muscle (*Figure 7.1*). The anterior neck contains the laryngeal skeleton — hyoid bone, thyroid cartilage and cricoid cartilage. The thyroid prominence (Adam's apple) is usually easily palpable and a good reference point.

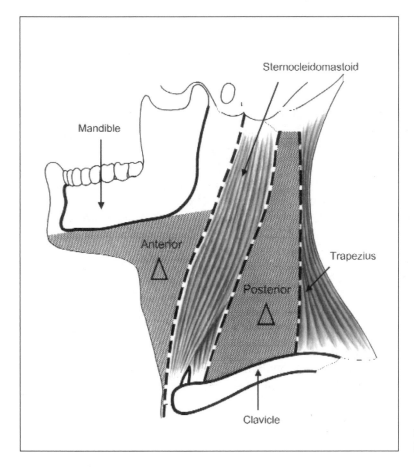

*Figure 7.1: Anatomical triangles in the neck.*

The position of lymph nodes involved in metastatic carcinoma is defined further by their description in a particular level (*Figure 7.2*). The level of a lymph node has been shown to be of prognostic relevance (Jones et al, 1994).

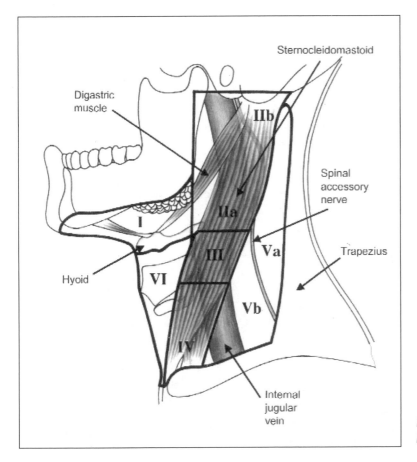

*Figure 7.2: Lymph node levels in the neck.*

The following definitions are recommended for the boundaries of cervical lymph node groups.

### Level I

Consists of the submental and submandibular lymph nodes within the triangle bounded by the anterior belly of the digastric, the hyoid bone, the posterior belly of digastric and the body of the mandible.

### Level II (upper deep cervical)

Consists of lymph nodes located around the upper third of the internal jugular vein and adjacent spinal accessory nerve extending from the level of the carotid bifurcation to the skull base. There is a recent recommendation to further subdivide this level into the area anterior to the accessory nerve (level IIa) and that posterior to the nerve (level IIb).

### Level III (mid deep cervical)

Consists of lymph nodes around the middle third of the internal jugular vein extending from the carotid bifurcation superiorly to the cricothyroid notch inferiorly.

### Level IV (lower deep cervical)

Consists of lymph nodes located around the lower third of the internal jugular vein extending from the cricothyroid notch to the clavicle inferiorly.

### Level V

Consists of the posterior triangle nodes, which are located between the posterior border of the sternomastoid muscle and the anterior border of trapezius. The supraclavicular nodes are also included in this group.

### Level VI

Anterior compartment.

## Reaching a diagnosis

The diagnosis is from the history, examination and investigations, including endoscopy, radiology and laboratory tests.

Symptoms of sore throat or upper respiratory tract infection may suggest an inflammatory cervical lymphadenopathy. Persistent hoarseness of voice, sore throat, pain on swallowing, cough or the sensation of a lump in the throat are risk symptoms of an upper aerodigestive tract malignancy. The symptoms are particularly relevant in patients who are over the age of 40 years and smoke cigarettes.

The anatomical position of the lump should be considered in context with the cervical viscera (e.g. parotid, thyroid gland, lymph nodes) that may be affected. The diagnosis is sometimes obvious from this evaluation, but it is dangerous to act impulsively on this limited information without establishing the diagnosis with relevant investigations. The patient should be referred promptly to an otolaryngologist who can examine the neck and upper aerodigestive tract. The specific investigations will then be dictated by the differential diagnosis.

# Investigations

## Open biopsy

The adverse effects of excisional or incisional biopsy as a primary diagnostic manoeuvre in the management of a neck lump are well documented in the literature. If the lump turns out to be a metastatic node from a squamous cell carcinoma, harm has been done to the patient. Open biopsy of a metastatic node, advanced age and nodal stage all have an adverse effect on survival (Jones et al, 1993; Janot et al, 1996). Open biopsy also makes subsequent examination of the neck more difficult, encourages fungation (*Figure 7.3*), increases the risk of subsequent recurrence in the neck and entails an unnecessary hospital admission and general anaesthetic for the patient (McGuirt and McCabe, 1978; Gooder and Palmer, 1984; Birchall et al, 1991).

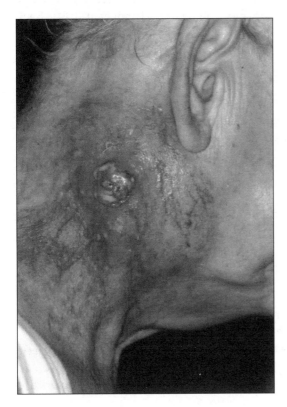

*Figure 7.3: A fungating neck lump. This patient had excision of a cystic neck lump that was subsequently discovered to be a squamous cell carcinoma. The patient was treated with postoperative radiotherapy. However, the disease recurred with typical fungation into the skin of the neck. Subsequent investigation confirmed a primary tumour in the ipsilateral tonsil, and treatment necessitated a combined oro-mandibular resection, radical neck dissection, wide excision of the involved skin and reconstruction.*

The dangers of performing an incisional or excisional biopsy (enucleation) in parotid tumours are now well known. In these circumstances the wound is inevitably seeded, and recurrence is likely. Recurrent disease may present late, involve the facial nerve or become malignant, and is exceptionally difficult to manage (Jackson et al, 1993).

There are occasions when fine-needle aspiration cytology (FNAC) and other investigations have failed to confirm the diagnosis, or have indicated a lesion whereupon excision or incision biopsy is required (e.g. suspected lymphoma, benign neck lump). However, it is recommended that this conclusion be reached after the patient has been examined by an otolaryngologist and undergone at least a diagnostic FNAC.

## Fine-needle aspiration cytology

The role of FNAC has been extensively evaluated. It offers an accurate, sensitive, inexpensive and rapid method for evaluation of a neck lump. Its use has been recommended in parotid lesions (Roland et al, 1994), thyroid disease and just about every other type of head and neck lump (Caslin et al, 1994). Immediate procurement in the clinic is possible and has the advantage of allowing the cytologist to repeat the procedure if an inadequate specimen is aspirated. In addition, it enables the clinician to inform the patient of the diagnosis, order other relevant investigations and make early management plans (Eisele et al, 1992; Caslin et al, 1994). For patients with poorly defined or deep-seated lesions, image or ultrasound guidance can be used (Righi et al, 1997; Sack et al, 1998).

FNAC is probably the single most useful diagnostic procedure if a neoplastic lymph node is suspected. False-negative and, rarely, false-positive results can occur with FNAC, so the information must always be used in conjunction with the clinical findings. Direct liaison between the clinician and cytologist is important. It has been said that FNAC is as accurate and reliable as the combined judgment of the clinician and cytologist. When there is diagnostic doubt, clinical judgment should always prevail. In a few cases an open biopsy may be the only method to determine the diagnosis.

## Radiology

An ultrasound scan (with ultrasound-guided FNAC) may delineate impalpable nodes. Ultrasound scanning (with ultrasound-guided FNAC) is the investigation of choice to define a thyroid nodule's position and nature.

Magnetic resonance imaging (MRI) may confirm the exact site and extent of a head and neck primary tumour. An MRI scan may also delineate impalpable nodes.

The scans can also reveal the integrity or involvement of the vasculature by a metastatic lymph node. In addition, an MRI scan is useful to identify the position and assess the size and vascularity of a carotid body tumour (a digital subtraction angiogram will enable precise delineation).

A chest radiograph may show a primary carcinoma or evidence of secondary spread, as well as pulmonary tuberculosis or mediastinal gland enlargement.

A barium swallow is useful in cases of suspected pharyngeal pouch, and may illustrate a carcinoma of the hypopharynx or cervical oesophagus.

For thyroglossal cysts, many experts recommend a $^{99m}$Tc or radioactive iodine ($^{131}$I) uptake scan before excision, although an ultrasound scan is less invasive, will delineate the cyst and will enable confirmation of whether there is a normal gland present.

Plain anteroposterior and lateral neck radiographs may show an air-filled sac (laryngocele).

Positron emission tomography is thought by some to have a place in the investigation of patients who have a primary of unknown origin.

### Laboratory tests

Laboratory tests have little role to play, but a full blood count may reveal a blood dyscrasia or high white cell count consistent with an infective cause of the lump. A raised erythrocyte sedimentation rate may occur in cases of inflammation, sarcoid or disseminated neoplasia. Human immunodeficiency virus testing may be appropriate, depending on the circumstances and index of suspicion.

## Conclusion

There are many causes of a neck lump in an adult, but management is dictated by the fact that a significant proportion may represent metastatic cervical lymphadenopathy. Upper aerodigestive tract examination and fine-needle aspiration biopsy are mandatory. Early referral to a surgeon with a specialist interest is advisable. Excisional or incisional biopsy is inadvisable and may be detrimental to the patient's care.

## References

Birchall MA, Stafford ND, Walsh-Waring GP (1991) Malignant neck lumps: a measured approach. *Ann R Coll Surg Engl* **73**: 91–5

Caslin A, Roland NJ, Turnbull L, Smith P, Jones A (1994) Immediate diagnosis of lesions of the head and neck by FNAC in outpatient clinics. *Clin Otolaryngol* **19**(3): 269

Eisele DW, Sherman ME, Koch WM, Richtsmeier WJ, Wu AY, Erozan YS (1992) Utility of immediate on-site cytopathological procurement and evaluation in fine needle aspiration. *Laryngoscope* **102**: 1328–30

Flanagan P, Roland NJ, Jones AS (1994) Cervical node metastases presenting with features of a branchial cyst. *J Otolaryngol* **108**: 1068–71

Gooder P, Palmer M (1984) Cervical lymph node biopsy — a study of its morbidity. *J Laryngol Otol* **98**: 1031–40

Jackson S, Roland NJ, Clarke R, Jones AS (1993) Recurrent pleomorphic adenoma. *J Laryngol Otol* **107**: 546–9

Janot F, Klijanienko J, Russo A et al (1996) Prognostic value of clinicopathological parameters in head and neck squamous cell carcinoma: a prospective analysis. *Br J Cancer* **73**(4): 531–8

Jones AS, Cook JA, Phillips D, Roland NJ (1993) Squamous carcinoma presenting as an enlarged cervical lymph node. *Cancer* **72**: 1756–61

Jones AS, Roland NJ, Field JK, Phillips DE (1994) The level of cervical node metastases: their prognostic relevance and relationship with head and neck squamous carcinoma primary sites. *Clin Otolaryngol* **19**: 63–9

McGuirt WF, McCabe BF (1978) Significance of node biopsy before definitive treatment of cervical metastatic carcinoma. *Laryngoscope* **88**: 594–7

Righi PD, Kopecky KK, Ball VA, Weisberger EC, Radour S (1997) Comparison of fine-needle aspiration and computed tomography in patients undergoing elective neck dissection. *Head Neck* **19**: 604–10

Roland NJ, Caslin A, Turnbull L, Smith P, Jones AS (1994) Fine-needle aspration cytology of salivary gland lesions reported immediately in a head and neck clinic. *J Laryngol Otol* **107**: 1025–8

Sack MJ, Weber RS, Weinstein GS, Chalain AA, Nisenbaum HI, Yousem DM (1998) Image-guided fine-needle aspiration of the head and neck: 5 year's experience. *Arch Otolaryngol Head Neck Surg* **124**: 1155–61

# Chapter 8

# Salivary gland stones: diagnosis and treatment

*Peter D Bull*

Salivary calculi are a common cause of salivary gland disorder and may occur in any of the salivary glands and at almost any age. The stones may be small and intraductal or lie within the gland substance, where they may become large. They cause symptoms by obstructing salivary flow. Diagnosis is usually straightforward, and treatment is aimed at stone removal.

While the aetiology of salivary stones is poorly understood, they are much more common in the submandibular than in the parotid gland (83% as opposed to 10%), with the remainder being in the minor salivary glands or the sublingual glands (Rauch, 1959). The reason for this is that the submandibular gland produces mucoid as well as serous saliva, allowing inspissation of the mucus to occur, particularly at times of dehydration or febrile illness. This then forms a nidus around which calcification can occur.

There appears to be no connection between the hardness of drinking water in an area and the incidence of salivary calculi in the population (Sherman and McGurk, 2000).

A Russian paper by Afanas'ev and Nikiforov (1999) suggested that a stricture in the duct might result in stasis and calculus formation. No metabolic cause of salivary stone formation has been demonstrated, although associations with diabetes and hypertension have been noted (Laforgia et al, 1989).

It has long been suspected that a small foreign body entering the salivary duct may act as a focus for stone formation, and Brophy (1916) demonstrated such detritus.

Saliva is saturated with hydroxyapatite, the basis of salivary stones. As a rule, acidic proteins in saliva will bind calcium and so prevent more frequent stone formation. Stones are ultimately formed by crystal formation from salivary solutes.

The structure of salivary calculi is that of progressive formation in layers around an organic nidus, usually with a laminar pattern. Riesco et al (1999) have shown an early sialolith from a minor salivary gland to have mineralized inclusion bodies, with calcium and phosphate being distributed in the outer coating of the stone.

Mature stones contain calcium phosphate in various crystalline forms associated with organic mucoprotein. Scanning electron microscopy has demonstrated concentric laminae (Taniguchi et al, 1979).

## Clinical features of salivary calculi

While some calculi may remain symptomless and are found incidentally, most declare themselves by obstruction of salivary outflow. This leads to painful enlargement of the affected gland, and if prolonged stasis ensues there will be subsequent infection.

The obstructed gland becomes tense and painful, usually during or immediately following a meal. Often the swelling subsides after an hour or so. If there is no associated infection there is no redness of the gland, but there will be marked tenderness.

Inspection of the relevant salivary duct may reveal the presence of an impacted stone. The salivary flow will usually be reduced or absent, but there is usually no inflammation of the duct opening unless the condition is chronic.

On bimanual examination of the submandibular duct, it may be possible to feel a stone, usually in the anterior third of the duct. Parotid stones are much smaller and softer and are more difficult to feel. Large stones may occur within the substance of a gland, usually the submandibular and only rarely the parotid. Here they may give rise to no symptoms and be found only because of a visible or palpable swelling, or incidentally on radiology.

## Natural history

Small calculi may discharge spontaneously from the duct, followed by a gush of turbid saliva (*Figure 8.1*). More usually, the stone in the duct will give rise to repeated episodes of duct obstruction and swelling. Ultimately, the gland will become atrophic and fibrosed (*Figure 8.2*), unless an acute abscess supervenes.

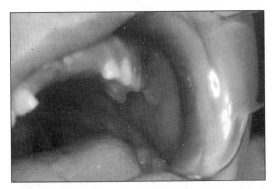

Figure 8.1: Turbid saliva oozing from the parotid duct.

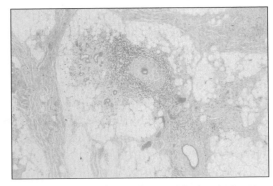

Figure 8.2: Histology of parotid gland showing chronic fibrosis and acinar atrophy.

The cost of treating symptomatic salivary stones has been calculated by Escudier and McGurk (1999). Based on an incidence of 27 per million population and possibly up to 59 per million population per year, a cost to the NHS of up to £4 million each year is suggested.

# Investigation

The aim of investigation is to determine whether a stone is present in the duct or gland. Biochemical investigation is unrewarding unless recurrent sialolithiasis suggests hypercalcaemia.

Lateral plain X-rays are poor at showing salivary gland calculi. Most parotid stones are radio-lucent, although 80–90% of submandibular stones contain calcium and so are visible on X-ray examination. It is preferable to take intra-oral views of both the submandibular and parotid ducts, which are more likely to show intraductal stones (*Figure 8.3*).

If the stone is thought to be in the body of the submandibular gland, lateral or oblique films will show its presence (*Figure 8.4*). Only rarely do large calculi occur in the parotid, and they are unlikely to be radio-opaque. Magnetic resonance (MR) scanning will reveal stones and can be combined with digital subtraction sialography (Heverhagen et al, 2000).

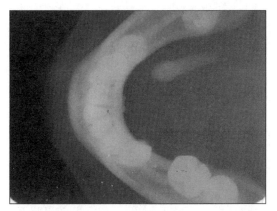

*Figure 8.3: Intra-oral view showing a large stone in the submandibular duct.*

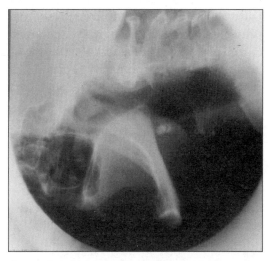

*Figure 8.4: Lateral view showing a stone within the submandibular gland.*

Ultrasound scanning is of limited value but may show a parotid ductal stone. Dense calculi may be revealed by acoustic shadowing deep to the stone. Because of its sensitivity to calcium salts, computed tomography (CT) scanning is accurate in finding calculi (Mandel and Hatzis, 2000) (*Figure 8.5*).

Sumi et al (1999) have described using MR and CT together as being complementary, and found that they may be more accurate when used in combination.

Endoscopy of the salivary ducts has been combined with endoscopic removal of salivary stones with a high rate of success and no major complications (Nahlieli and Baruchin, 1997).

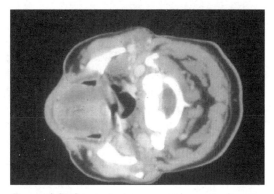

*Figure 8.5: Computed tomography scan showing a stone within the left parotid gland.*

## Treatment of sialolithiasis

The treatment of salivary calculi is determined by the symptoms and the position of the stone.

A symptomless stone found incidentally by clinical examination or radiology will usually require no treatment. A stone within the submandibular duct causing intermittent obstruction can usually be removed by the intra-oral route. If such a stone cannot be seen or felt, it will be difficult to remove. Similarly, a stone at the distal end of the parotid duct can be removed intra-orally.

A large stone within the submandibular gland or at the hilum will necessitate excision of the submandibular gland. Similarly, a stone deep within the ductal system of the parotid gland (*Figure 8.6*) will require parotidectomy. The surgery for these procedures has been described by Bull and Bath (1997). The overriding consideration is the avoidance of nerve damage. In parotid surgery, it is primarily the facial nerve that is at risk, while operations on the submandibular gland hazard the marginal mandibular branch of the facial nerve, the lingual nerve, which is intimately related to the submandibular duct, and the hypoglossal nerve if the gland is enlarged.

Removal of salivary calculi by a wire basket extractor under radiological control has been described (Drage et al, 2000). It is most effective in removing stones from the extraglandular duct of either the parotid or submandibular gland.

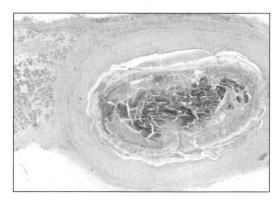

*Figure 8.6: A calculus within the parotid duct (operative specimen).*

Extracorporeal shock wave lithotripsy has been described by Iro et al (1998) with encouraging results.

## Surgical technique for removing a stone from the submandibular duct

The operation can be performed either under local or general anaesthetic. The mouth is opened widely and the calculus identified (*Figure 8.7*). Infiltration with local anaesthetic with added adrenaline (epinephrine) will reduce bleeding. A stay suture is passed around the duct proximal to the stone to prevent the stone slipping back. If the stone can be felt easily, a longitudinal incision

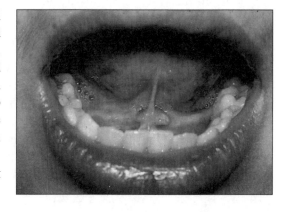

*Figure 8.7: A stone at the orifice of the left submandibular duct.*

over the calculus is made and the stone extracted (*Figure 8.8*). If the stone is more difficult to identify, the duct must be dissected and demonstrated, so that it can be opened. It can also be opened from its orifice, and the calculi milked forward. No attempt at closure of the duct is made. The position of the lingual nerve (sensory to the anterior two-thirds of the tongue) must be considered and nerve damage avoided.

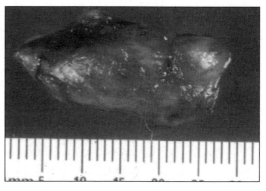

*Figure 8.8: The stone removed from the submandibular duct in Figure 8.3.*

Complications include residual stones, ranula (retention cyst) in the floor of the mouth (*Figure 8.9*) and impairment of lingual nerve function.

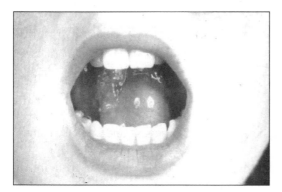

*Figure 8.9: A submandibular ranula following duct surgery.*

## Conclusion

While salivary stones are not life-threatening, their correct recognition and management are important in the avoidance of long-term morbidity and operative complications. New techniques, such as lithotripsy and endoscopy, hold promise of a safe means of treatment in the future.

## References

Afanas'ev VV, Nikiforov VS (1999) The etiology of salivary calculi. *Stomatologiia* **78**(5): 39–41

Brophy TW (1916) *Oral Surgery: A Treatise on the Diseases, Injuries and Malformations of the Mouth and Associated Parts*. Henry Kimpton, London

Bull PD, Bath AP (1997) Technique and indications of salivary gland surgery. *Surgery* **15**(9): 205–10

Drage NA, Brown JE, Escudier M, McGurk M (2000) Interventional radiology in the removal of salivary calculi. *Radiology* **214**(1): 139–42

Escudier MP, McGurk M (1999) Symptomatic sialoadenitis and sialolithiasis in the English population, an estimate of the cost of hospital treatment. *Br Dent J* **186**(9): 463–6

Heverhagen JT, Kalinowski M, Rehberg E, Klose KJ, Wagner HJ (2000) Prospective comparison of magnetic resonance sialography and digital subtraction sialography. *J Magn Reson Imaging* **11**(5): 518–24

Iro H, Zenk J, Waldfahrer F, Benzel W, Schneider T, Ell C (1998) Extracorporeal shock wave lithotripsy of parotid stones. Results of a prospective clinical trial. *Ann Otol Rhinol Laryngol* **107**(10 I): 860–4

Laforgia PD, Favia GF, Chiaravalle N, Lacaita MG, Laforgia A (1989) Clinico-statistical, morphologic and microstructural analysis of 400 cases of sialolithiasis. *Minerva Stomatol* **38**: 1329–36

Mandel L, Hatzis G (2000) The role of computerised tomography in the diagnosis and treatment of parotid stones: a case report. *J Am Dent Assoc* **131**(4): 479–82

Nahlieli O, Baruchin AM (1997) Sialoendoscopy — 3 years' experience as a diagnostic and treatment modality. *J Oral Maxillofac Surg* **55**(9): 912–18

Rauch S (1959) *Die Speicheldrüsen des Menschen*. Thieme, Stuttgart

Riesco JM, Juanes JA, Diaz-Gonzalez M, Blanco EJ, Riesco-Lopez JM, Vazquez R (1999) Crystalloid architecture of a sialolith in a minor salivary gland. *J Oral Pathol Med* **28**(10): 451–5

Sherman JA, McGurk M (2000) Lack of correlation between water hardness and salivary calculi in England. *Br J Oral Maxillofac Surg* **38**(1): 50–3

Sumi M, Izumi M, Yonetsu K, Nakamura T (1999) The MR imaging assessment of submandibular gland sialoadenitis secondary to sialolithiasis: correlation with CT and histopathologic findings. *Am J Neuroradiol* **20**(9): 1737–43

Taniguchi T, Yamamoto S, Yamada S, Ohyama M (1979) Scanning electron microscopic X-ray microanalytical studies of salivary calculi. *Otol Fukuoka* **25**(suppl 5): 757

# Chapter 9

# Benign salivary gland disease

*PJ Bradley*

Most benign clinical problems that present affect the major salivary glands — parotid and submandibular. However, there are numerous minor salivary glands located in the mucosa of the head and neck, which have the same predilection to the same diseases that affect the major glands but to a lesser frequency.

There are many different conditions that affect the salivary glands. A working classification to be considered in this chapter is inflammatory and non-inflammatory conditions. This group of disorders can afflict the major salivary glands (the parotid and submandibular) and the minor salivary glands (the sublingual), which are mainly concentrated in the oral cavity. These conditions are generally much more common in the major glands. Both adults and children are affected, and the reader is directed to a review of some of the uncommon conditions that may specifically affect children (Bradley, 1997).

This chapter updates the reader on the current state of knowledge regarding the common inflammatory and non-inflammatory conditions that may present both in the adult and the child.

## Inflammatory conditions

### Acute viral inflammatory lesions

The most common viral disorder involving the salivary glands is mumps (infectious parotitis), and it is probably the most common cause of parotid swelling. The peak incidence of mumps as a contagious infectious disease is in 4–6-year-olds. The incubation period is 2–3 weeks, which leads to pain and swelling accompanied by fever, malaise, myalgia and headache. The diagnosis is made by demonstrating antibodies to the mumps S and V antigens and to the haemagglutination antigen. More than 95% of adults have neutralizing antibodies. Major complications are uncommon, but include pancreatitis, meningitis, sudden deafness and orchitis.

Other viral agents also affect the salivary glands and mimic the mumps signs. They include coxsackie A, enteric cytopathic human orphan (ECHO) viruses, influenza A, lymphocytic choriomeningitis and cytomegalovirus. The treatment for viral infections is symptomatic.

### Acute suppurative sialadenitis

The parotid gland is most commonly involved in acute suppurative sialadenitis. This increased parotid susceptibility is believed to be the result of the lessened bacteriostatic activity of the saliva produced by the parotid when compared with that of the submandibular gland. Acute suppurative sialadenitis accounts for 0.03% of hospital admissions, with 30–40% of these occurring in postoperative patients. The disease typically commences postoperatively on days 3–5, with the highest incidence after gastrointestinal procedures. It occurs in approximately one per 1000–2000 procedures, and is usually associated with dehydration. Patients aged 50–70 years are the most frequently affected, with equal sex distribution. Predisposing factors include calculi, duct stricture and dehydration, coupled with poor oral hygiene.

The usual presentation is the sudden onset of diffuse enlargement of the involved gland with associated tenderness, induration and pain. Purulent saliva can be seen at the duct orifice, particularly with massage of the gland. The saliva can occasionally culture coagulase-positive *Staphylococcus aureus* with other aerobic organisms, particularly *Streptococcus pneumoniae*, *Escherichia coli* and *Haemophilus influenzae*. Approximately 20% of infections are bilateral.

Initial treatment includes adequate hydration, improved oral hygiene, repeated massage of the gland and intravenous antibiotics. The empirical administration of a penicillinase-resistant anti-staphylococcal antibiotic should be started while awaiting the culture results. Dramatic improvements should ensue within the first 24–48 hours. If not, incision and drainage should be considered. Fluctuation within the parotid gland does not occur until late in the course of the disease because of the multiple investing fascia within the gland. The abscess can be located using ultrasound or computerized tomography (CT) scanning.

## Chronic inflammatory disorders

The key causative event in chronic sialadenitis is thought to be a lowered secretion rate with subsequent salivary stasis (Bhatty et al, 1998). Chronic sialadenitis is more common in the parotid gland than in the submandibular gland. It may occasionally affect the minor salivary glands, most commonly in the lower lip. This condition may result in permanent damage to the glandular ductal system because of the acute or chronic suppuration. Persisting damage, with time, may be a sequelae to sialectasis, ductal ectasia and progressive acinar destruction combined with a lymphocytic infiltrate. The sialographical appearance parallels the degree of histological damage.

In such patients, there is generally a history of mildly painful recurrent parotid enlargement, aggravated by eating. The clinician should look for treatable predisposing factors, such as a calculus or stricture. If no treatable cause is found, the patient management should be conservative and include the use of sialagogues, frequent gland massages and antibiotics for acute exacerbations. Should conservative measures fail, other treatments include periodic duct dilatation, ligation of the duct, total gland irradiation, tympanic neurectomy (Daud and Pahor, 1995) and excision of the gland. Only the excision of the gland works uniformly.

Chronic recurrent parotitis may eventually lead to the development of a benign lymphoepithelial lesion. This lesion belongs in the spectrum of diseases characterized by a lymphoreticular infiltrate combined with acinar atrophy and ductal metaplasia. The ductal metaplasia ends in the development of epimyoepithelial islands. This lesion is first noticed as an asymptomatic enlargement, unless there is associated infection. If the lesion becomes cosmetically unacceptable, excision of the gland may be necessary (Carlson, 2000). There are well-documented cases of the evolution of this disease into more aggressive entities, including lymphoproliferative disorders, carcinoma (undifferentiated type) and pseudolymphoma (Nagao et al, 1983). The lymphoproliferative disorders are usually non-Hodgkin's lymphomas involving the extrasalivary sites.

# Granulomatous diseases

### Primary tuberculosis

Primary tuberculosis is unusual. The disease is usually unilateral, and the parotid gland is the most frequently involved salivary gland. It is believed to spread from a focus of infection in the tonsils or the teeth. It can present in one of two ways:

- an acute inflammatory lesion
- chronic tumorous lesion.

Often the diagnosis is not made until an acid-fast salivary stain and a purified protein derivative (PPD) skin test are performed. The PPD test may be unreliable because the infection may be caused by atypical mycobacteria and may produce a negative skin test (Ganesan et al, 2000). The treatment is as for any acute tuberculous infection (Kanlikama et al, 2000).

### Animal scratch disease

Animal scratch disease does not involve the salivary glands directly, but may involve the periparotid and submandibular triangle lymph nodes, and these may involve the salivary glands by contiguous spread. Cat scratch disease is one such entity, which primarily involves children and young adults. A history of animal contact, usually cats or even kittens (scratches, bites or even licks by a cat), has been elicited in 67–90% of reported cases. Recently, the true origin of this disease has been implicated as *Bartonella henselae*, a Gram-negative bacterium. A polymerase chain reaction assay to detect bartonella DNA has been used to identify the agent. A serology test for patients with cat scratch disease has shown titres of at least 1:64 for *B. henselae* antibodies (Malatskey et al, 2000). Treatment consists of supportive therapy and reassurance, as antibiotics have not been shown to be effective in shortening the course of the disease. The lymphadenopathy usually disappears within 2–3 months without complications.

# Sarcoidosis

Clinically, salivary gland involvement occurs in only 6% of cases. Uveoparotid fever (Heerfordt's disease) is a particular form of sarcoidosis characterized by uveitis, parotid enlargement and facial palsy. It usually occurs in 20–30-year-olds. The swelling can last from months to years without suppuration, but will eventual resolve.

### Sjögren's syndrome

Sjögren's syndrome is a common disorder, which occurs predominantly in women (9 females:1 male) in the fourth and fifth decades of life, with the correct diagnosis often being made a few years after the initial clinical presentation.

At present, there is no single definitive test that accurately diagnoses Sjögren's syndrome, and therefore several sets of diagnostic criteria have been proposed (Sood et al, 2000):

* Enlargement of one or more of the major salivary glands may occur and is usually self-limiting.
* Parotid swelling is more common than submandibular gland swelling and may be recurrent and painful.
* Lymphoma is an important complication, with an estimated relative risk for developing lymphoma in patients with Sjögren's syndrome of between 33–44%.
* The presence of serum autoantibodies to Ro (SS-A) or La (SS-B) antigens, antinuclear antibodies or rheumatoid factor with clinical signs and symptoms helps with diagnosis.

Treatment is empirical (Tzioufas and Moutsopoulos, 1998).

# Sialolithiasis

Eighty per cent of salivary calculi occur in the submandibular gland, with the remaining 19% occurring in the parotid gland and approximately 1% in the sublingual gland. In 75% of cases, only a single stone is found. Gout is the only systemic disease known to be associated with salivary calculi, and these stones are composed of uric acid. The majority of calculi seen and diagnosed are calcium phosphate with small amounts of magnesium, ammonia and carbonate. Despite their similar chemical make up, 90% of submandibular calculi are radio-opaque, whereas 90% of parotid calculi are radiolucent (Bodner, 1999).

The theoretical cause for the formation of stones or calculi is some anatomical nidus of precipitate calcium material, which is associated with saliva fluid stasis. The submandibular gland is considered more susceptible to sialolithiasis than the other salivary glands because its saliva is more alkaline and has a higher concentration of calcium and phosphate, coupled with a higher mucin content. The duct is longer and flows a distance of several centimeters, from the gland at the back of the mouth to the front of the mouth where it opens.

Most patients present with a history of recurrent swelling and pain in the gland, which is usually aggravated by eating. The calculus may be palpable in the duct, and the involved gland is swollen and tender. Occlusal plain X-rays of the floor of the mouth frequently reveal the stone in the submandibular duct or gland, but are less reliable in the parotid gland. Sialography is essentially 100% effective in making the diagnosis, but can be complemented with CT scanning. The complications of sialolithiasis include acute suppurative sialadenitis, ductal ectasia and stricture.

Treatment depends on the location of the calculus: simple ductoplasty can be used to remove the stone if it is visualized or palpated anteriorly in the anterior floor of the mouth near the duct opening or papilla. If the stone is located more distally in the duct or located near the gland itself, excision of the submandibular gland is indicated. The use of extracorporeal shock-wave lithotripsy may be useful in the management of parotid calculus to minimize resultant cosmetic deformity (Iro et al, 1998). Simple removal of the stone is associated with a recurrence of the stone in about 18% of cases, as the underlying cause, which may be unknown, may not be corrected.

# Non-inflammatory

## Cystic lesions

True cysts of the parotid gland account for less than 5% of lesions presenting. The cysts may be either acquired or congenital. Type I branchial arch cysts are a duplication anomaly of the membraneous external auditary canal (Arndal and Bonding, 1996), whereas type II cysts are a duplication anomaly of the membraneous and cartilaginous external auditary canal. Excision during a quiescent period with preservation of the facial nerve is curative.

Acquired cysts may be associated with mucus extravasation, parotitis, trauma, calculi, ductal obstruction, benign epithelial lesions and neoplasms (Antoniadis et al, 1990). If the cyst is associated with a salivary duct stenosis, correcting or fixing the stenosis may cure the cystic swelling by encouraging drainage. Should this treatment not be possible or attempts to treat it have failed, the cystic lesion itself should be excised. Some cysts that present may not be of the 'simple' variety, but may be associated with neoplasms, such as pleomorphic adenoma, adenoid cystic carcinoma, mucoepidermoid carcinoma and Warthin's tumour. There is a special type of cystic lesion found in the floor of the mouth. This is the mucus retention cyst or ranula of the sublingual gland, which is visible from the neck because of its size and therefore called 'the plunging ranula' (Davison et al, 1998). The treatment is excision.

### *Sialadenosis*

Sialadenosis is a non-specific term used to describe a non-inflammatory, non-neoplastic enlargement of a salivary gland, usually the parotid (Pape et al, 1995). The enlargement is generally asymptomatic, and the mechanism of aetiology is unknown in many cases. Bilateral parotid enlargement is common in obesity, secondary to fatty hypertrophy. Complete endocrine and metabolic screening should be performed before making this diagnosis. Diagnoses such as diabetes mellitus, hypertension, hyperlipidaemia and menopause are associated. This condition has also been associated with alcoholic cirrhosis; it is rare in non-alcoholic cirrhosis. The prognosis is good if the underlying disease can be corrected. Sometimes surgical excision is indicated to correct the cosmetic deformity.

## Salivary gland neoplasms

The neoplasms that arise in the major and minor salivary glands can be benign or malignant in nature. They may also be the source of primary salivary malignant or secondary malignant neoplasms.

The prevalence of primary salivary neoplasms is estimated to be more common in the parotid gland than in the other glands. The distribution by site follows the 100:10:1:10 rule for the proportions of salivary tumours in the four main sites; benign to malignant salivary tumours are more frequently found in the parotid gland than in the other sites (*Table 9.1*).

**Table 9.1: Prevalence of population-based study of benign and malignant salivary gland neoplasms (Bradley, 2001a)**

|  | Prevalence | Benign (%) | Malignant (%) |
|---|---|---|---|
| **Major salivary glands** | | | |
| Parotid | 100 | 84 | 16 |
| Submandibular | 10 | 61 | 39 |
| Sublingual | 1 | 0 | 100 |
| **Minor salivary glands** | 10 | 64 | 36 |

The incidence of malignant salivary neoplasms was found to be 0.8 per 100 000 population, and of benign salivary neoplasms to be 7.2 per 100 000 population in a Nottingham population over a 10-year period (Bradley, 2001a). In most populations worldwide it is difficult to estimate the true incidence of benign salivary neoplastic disease because the condition is not registered, hence any figures are population based. Most benign neoplasms are adenomas – pleomorphic adenoma or adenolymphoma.

Benign neoplasms of the salivary glands are most frequently encountered in the parotid gland as a discrete lump in the salivary tissue. Serious consideration needs to be given to patients who present with a lump in a salivary gland as its history may not be typical, associated with fluctuation in size, tenderness and even pain, which may suggest a benign or inflammatory diagnosis. All such lumps must be investigated, and if a firm diagnosis cannot be made then the lump should be removed and examined by a pathologist to confirm the true nature of the disease.

Currently, with the changing pattern of disease presenting early, the sensitivity and specificity of clinical diagnosis can no longer be relied upon, and the investigation of choice for salivary gland neoplasms is fine-needle aspiration cytology (FNAC) and a CT scan. Should the FNAC be inconclusive, it is the opinion of the author that all patients with a suspected salivary neoplasm should be recommended for surgical removal.

It is agreed that the management of salivary gland neoplasms is surgical. Complete excision should be achieved; extracapsular excision is the goal, preserving preoperative intact neurological functions and minimising cosmetic defects. In the parotid gland, most lesions are located lateral to the facial nerve. Occasionally, the benign neoplasm is located deep to the nerve or located in the parapharyngeal space. Treatment remains surgical in these deeper locations, with preservation of the facial nerve. Should the tumour be incompletely excised, there remains a real risk that the tumour can recur and occasionally may metastasize (Bradley, 2005). The management of such patients who present with recurrent disease currently remains controversial (Bradley, 2001b).

## Other conditions

Parotid gland enlargement frequently occurs in patients with human immunodeficiency virus (HIV) infection (Huang et al, 1991). It usually occurs as a diffuse, symmetrical enlargement of both parotid glands, with or without involvement of the submandibular glands. This clinical presentation in a young patient should raise the suspicion of HIV infection. In such a patient, a CT scan is recommended to aid diagnosis and location of the associated cystic lesions. The additional use of FNAC of the cyst fluid and confirmation that the fluid contains amylase will confirm the diagnosis of HIV. Watchful waiting is advised for such cytic pathology.

## Conclusion

Inflammatory and non-inflammatory conditions, including salivary neoplasms, may present with similar clinical histories and physical findings, both in adults and children. An accurate diagnosis is essential to optimize patient management, to minimize the likelihood of chronicity and to offer patients a prognosis. It is current best practice to perform a needle biopsy on all discrete masses that persist for >2 months, when such a lesion persists in the parotid and submandibular glands. Diffuse swellings of the major salivary glands are a more difficult clinical challenge and should be referred to a specialist. To assume that a local diagnosis of a benign disease is all that is necessary in salivary glands, and not to consider serious or systemic disease, may result in serious patient mismanagement.

# References

Antoniadis K, Karakasis D, Tzarou V, Skordalaki A (1990) Benign cysts of the parotid. *Int J Oral Maxillofac Surg* **19**: 139–40

Arndal H, Bonding P (1996) First branchial cleft anomaly. *Clin Otolaryngol* **21**: 203–7

Bhatty MA, Piggot TA, Soames JV, McClean NR (1998) Chronic non-specific parotid sialadenitis. *Br J Plastic Surg* **51**: 517–21

Bodner L (1999) Parotid sialolithiasis. *J Laryngol Otol* **113**: 266–7

Bradley PJ (1997) Salivary gland disorders in children. In: Cinnamond M, Adams D, eds. *Scott–Brown's Diseases of the Ear, Nose and Throat*. Vol 6. Paediatrics. Butterworth-Heinemann Ltd, Oxford: 1–14

Bradley PJ (2001a) General epidemiology and statistics in a defined UK population. In: McGurk M, Renehan A, eds. *Controversies in the Management of Salivary Gland Disease*. Oxford University Press, Oxford: 3–12

Bradley PJ (2001b) Recurrent salivary gland pleomorphic adenoma: aetiology, management and results. *Curr Opin Otolaryngol Head Neck Surg* **9**: 100–8

Bradley PJ (2005) 'Metastasizing pleomorphic salivary adenoma' should now be considered a low-grade malignancy with a lethal potential. *Curr Opin Otolaryngol Head Neck Surg* **13**: 123–6

Carlson GW (2000) The salivary glands: embryology, anatomy and surgical applications. *Surg Clin North Am* **80**(1): 261–73

Daud AS, Pahor AL (1995) Tympanic neurectomy in the management of parotid sialectasis. *J Laryngol Otol* **109**: 1155–8

Davison MJ, Morton RP, McIvor NP (1998) Plunging ranula: clinical observations. *Head and Neck* **20**: 63–8

Ganesan S, Thirwall A, Brewis C, Grant HR, Novelli VM (2000) Dual infection with atypical mycobacteria and *Mycobacterium tuberculosis* causing cervical lymphadenopathy in a child. *J Laryngol Otol* **114**: 649–51

Huang RD, Pearlman S, Friedman WH, Loree T (1991) Benign cystic versus solid lesions of the parotid gland in HIV patients. *Head and Neck* **13**: 522–7

Iro H, Zenk J, Waldfahrer F, Benzel W, Schneider T, Ell C (1998) Extracorporeal shock wave lithotripsy of parotid stones. *Ann Otol Rhinol Laryngol* **117**: 860–4

Kanlikama M, Mubuc S, Bayazit Y, Sirikci A (2000) Management strategy of mycobacterial cervical lymphadenitis. *J Laryngol Otol* **114**: 274–8

Malatskey S, Fradis M, Ben-David J, Podoshin L (2000) Cat-scratch disease of the parotid gland: an often-misdiagnosed entity. *Ann Otol Rhinol Laryngol* **109**: 676–82

Nagao K, Matsuzaki O, Saiga H et al (1983) A histopathologic study of benign and malignant lymphoepithelial lesions of the parotid. *Cancer* **52**: 1044–52

Pape SA, MacLeod RI, McLean NR, Soames JV (1995) Sialadenosis of the salivary glands. *Br J Plastic Surg* **48**: 419–22

Sood S, Anthony R, Pease CT (2000) Sjogrens Syndrome. *Clin Otolaryngol* **25**: 350–7

Tzioufas AG, Moutsopoulos HM (1998) Sjogren's syndrome. In: Kuppic JM, Dieppe PA, eds. *Rheumatology*. 2nd edn. Mosby International, London: 1–12

# Chapter 10

# Management of malignant salivary gland tumours

*ED Vaughan*

Malignant tumours of both major and minor salivary glands are extremely rare: the parotid gland is most frequently affected by malignant change, followed by the submandibular gland. Malignant tumours of minor salivary glands may occur anywhere in the upper aerodigestive tract, but more common sites are the upper lip, junction of hard and soft palate and paranasal sinuses.

Malignant salivary gland tumours account for 5.5% of head and neck cancers and represent 0.14% of all cancers. The majority occur in the parotid gland, accounting for 20% of all parotid masses, with mucoepidermoid carcinomas being the predominant malignant type.

In the submandibular gland, approximately 50% of submandibular masses are malignant, with adenoidcystic carcinomas being the most common type (40%). In the minor salivary glands, the commonest tumours include mucoepidermoid carcinomas and adenoidcystic carcinomas, and are extremely rare with approximately six cases being seen annually in Merseyside, which has a population of 2.2 million people.

## Aetiology

The cause of malignant change in salivary tissue is unknown. However, there is strong histological evidence of benign pleomorphic adenomas undergoing malignant transformation to carcinoma ex-pleomorphic adenoma. It has been estimated that the risk of malignant transformation is 20% over 30 years, according to Hollander and Cunningham (1973).

It would appear that there is no substance to the claims of an association with breast cancer (Bigger et al, 1983).

The role of radiation in the aetiology of malignant salivary gland disease is confused, with a reported increased incidence following high-dose exposure to radiation. However, no significant difference was reported in a series compiled by Watkin and Hobsley (1986).

## Clinical presentation

In most cases, malignant tumours present as painless, asymptomatic lumps in the substance of the parotid or submandibular gland (*Figure 10.1*). Generally speaking, the patients are usually in the 50–60-year-old age group, with mucoepidermoid carcinomas particularly affecting children.

Facial paresis as a presenting symptom is uncommon (*Figure 10.2*), tends to carry a poorer prognosis and occurs in approximately 8–33% of cases, depending on the type of tumour. Again, pain is an uncommon feature and should not be considered pathognomic of malignant disease.

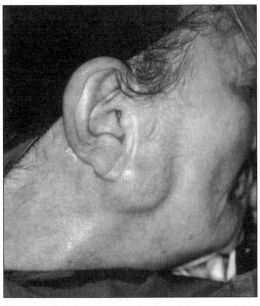

*Figure 10.1: Asymptomatic parotid mass, which was malignant histologically.*

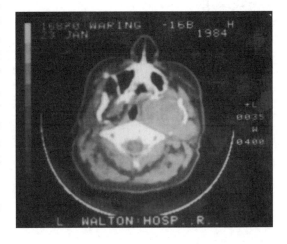

*Figure 10.2: Facial paresis as a presenting symptom of malignant tumours.*

Change in the rate of growth, with sudden increase in size, is considered by some to indicate malignant change. However, this feature occurs as commonly with benign tumours as with malignant tumours. Generally speaking, should the tumour be located in the deep lobe of the parotid gland, it will be larger and have infiltrated further before being diagnosed, as a result of the loose areolar tissue present. It may present with distortion of the lateral pharyngeal wall or soft palate on intra-oral examination (*Figure 10.3*).

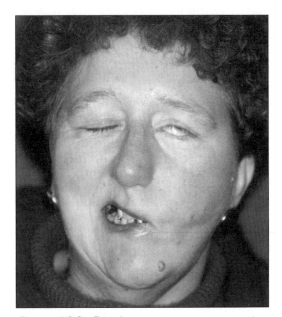

*Figure 10.3: Axial computed tomography scan of deep lobe parotid tumour.*

Trismus and pain in the distribution of the second and third divisions of the trigeminal nerve are worrying signs of infiltration within the infra-temporal fossa.

Overt involvement of the cervical lymph nodes is uncommon and denotes high-grade, advanced disease. However, 20% of cases have histological evidence of nodal involvement (Ball and Meirion Thomas, 1995).

In the case of minor salivary gland malignant neoplasms, presentation depends on the anatomical position of the tumour, with oral lesions presenting as non-tender sessile swellings, which may have a pink, red or blue appearance depending on the amount of mucoid material contained within the tumour (*Figure 10.4*). In time, the surface becomes ulcerated and secondarily infected (*Figure 10.5*).

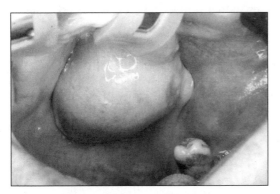

*Figure 10.4: Oral lesion presenting as non-tender sessile swelling.*

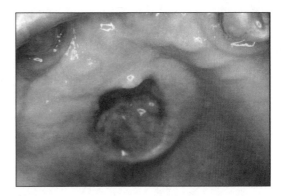

*Figure 10.5: Ulcerated surface of oral lesion.*

Tumours arising in the floor of the mouth may become quite large, because of the laxity of the soft tissues there. Clinically, if the location is sino-antral, it may be difficult to distinguish common squamous cell carcinoma from symptoms related to the mouth, including loose teeth or persistence of an oro-antral fistula from tooth extraction. If there is involvement of the nasal cavity, unilateral nasal obstruction and epistaxis are not uncommon but tend to be late features.

Other late manifestations include swelling of the cheek and loss of sensation in the distribution of the infra-orbital nerve. If the tumour extends upwards, orbital and ocular symptoms may predominate, with proptosis, epiphora and diplopia.

## Investigations

There are some who propose that preoperative knowledge of the histological type of tumour is irrelevant to the surgical treatment subsequently provided; this school of thought carries out no initial investigations (Spiro, 1986).

Others, on the other hand, attempt to determine the histological nature of the tumour before definitive surgery. They also attempt to define the location and extent of the lesion by radiological means in the hope that the acquisition of such knowledge will enable them to decide whether radical surgical treatment is appropriate.

For major salivary gland lesions, fine-needle aspiration (FNA) has become the preferred method of determining histology and is totally dependent on the skill of the cytopathologist. In skilled hands, an accuracy of over 90% may be expected.

In cases where there are clinical signs highly suggestive of malignancy, a 'tru-cut' needle biopsy may be performed, taking care to place the needle track in a position where it may be subsequently excised.

Both computed tomography and magnetic resonance scanning are extremely useful in delineating the extent of the tumour, and in many cases with a skilled radiologist it is possible to distinguish benign lesions from malignant ones.

For minor salivary gland tumours, one can, with varying degrees of ease and depending on location, perform an incisional biopsy with little or no risk of seeding of malignant cells.

Finally, if at the time of surgery the clinical appearance of the tumour gives rise to the suspicion of malignancy, it is appropriate to obtain a frozen section, providing one is confident of the ability of the pathologist to distinguish malignant disease from benign disease in this notoriously histologically difficult tissue.

## Treatment

The current consensus in treating malignant salivary gland neoplasms is for primary surgery to eradicate the tumour locally in three dimensions, while maintaining function where at all possible. Depending on the histological type and the adequacy of surgery, postoperative radiotherapy may be required.

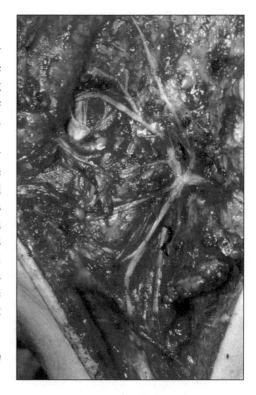

In the case of the parotid gland, this generally means a preservation of the facial nerve and the removal of the entire superficial lobe of the parotid gland (*Figure 10.6*). If at the time of surgery there is obvious infiltration of branches of the facial nerve, a decision has to be made whether or not it is appropriate to sacrifice these branches. The general view is that sacrificing branches of the facial nerve is a manoeuvre of last resort, and in most cases one should rely on postoperative radiotherapy to prevent local recurrence (Jackson et al, 1983).

*Figure 10.6: Preservation of facial nerve following superficial parotidectomy.*

Having performed a superficial parotidectomy with preservation of the facial nerve, should the tumour involve the deep lobe of the parotid gland it may be necessary to gain access to the infra-temporal fossa by a variety of means.

### Via a cervical approach

One usually combines the cervical approach (*Figure 10.7*) with some form of neck-clearing procedure, and access is obtained to the lower and posterior aspects of the infra-temporal fossa.

### Via a mandibulotomy

Access is gained (*Figure 10.8*) to the anterior aspect of the infra-temporal fossa.

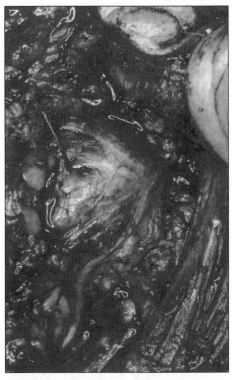

Figure 10.7: Cervical approach — tumour deep to branches of the facial nerve.

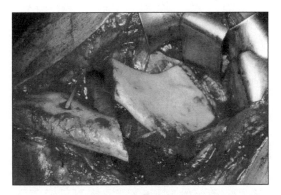

Figure 10.8: Access to antero-inferior aspect of infra-temporal fossa.

### Via a mid-face approach (Altemir)

This approach (*Figure 10.9*) will allow access to the roof and anterior aspects of the infra-temporal fossa.

Figure 10.9: Mid-face approach to the infra-temporal fossa.

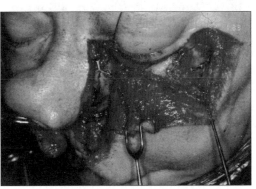

### Via a subtemporal approach

In this approach (*Figure 10.10*), the zygomatic bone is removed and allows access to the roof of the infra-temporal fossa.

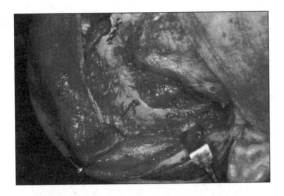

*Figure 10.10: Subtemporal approach to the infra-temporal fossa.*

### Via a mandibulectomy approach

Access is gained to virtually the entire infra-temporal fossa (*Figure 10.11*).

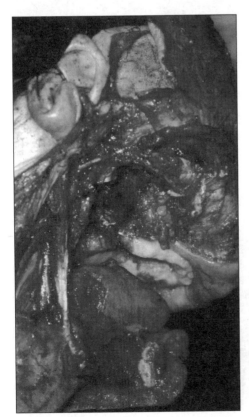

*Figure 10.11: Mandibulectomy to access the infra-temporal fossa.*

In high-grade tumours, where there is no possibility of preserving the facial nerve, it is appropriate to sacrifice the facial nerve and, if necessary, the overlying skin (*Figure 10.12*).

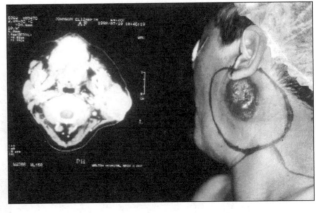

*Figure 10.12: High-grade tumours may require sacrifice of the facial nerve and overlying skin.*

The resultant facial nerve defect is reconstructed with either a vascularized or non-vascularized radial nerve graft harvested from the non-dominant forearm (*Figure 10.13*).

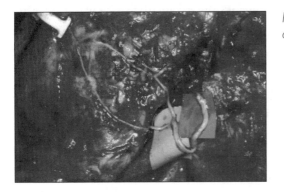

*Figure 10.13: Reconstructing a facial nerve defect with a radial nerve graft.*

The graft may be combined with a fascio cutaneous-free radial forearm flap (*Figure 10.14*).

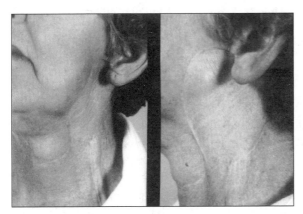

*Figure 10.14: Graft combined with a fascio cutaneous-free radial forearm flap.*

The results of such reconstructions are acceptable, even when postoperative radiotherapy has been employed (*Figure 10.15a,b,c*) (Jackson et al, 1983; Vaughan and Richardson, 1993).

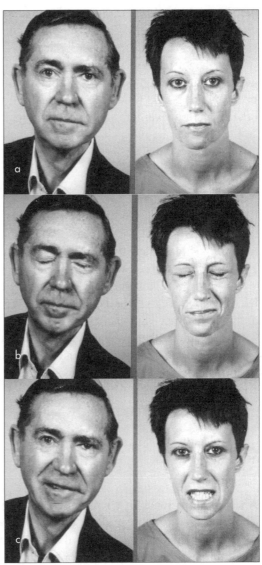

*Figure 10.15: Facial nerve reconstruction in terms of (a) facial symmetry, (b) eye closure and (c) ability to smile.*

## Neck dissection

The role of neck dissection in the management of malignant salivary gland disease is not clear. In the case of an asymptomatic parotid swelling that subsequently proves to be malignant, the factor that will decide whether it is appropriate to perform a neck dissection will be the histological type. In the case of high-grade mucoepidermoid and adenoid cystic carcinomas, carcinoma ex-pleomorphic adenoma and other adenocarcinomas, it would be reasonable to perform a selective function-preserving neck dissection, to include levels I–V secondarily.

Where there are obvious signs of malignancy and where there are involved neck nodes, again a selective neck dissection should be performed in continuity with the primary resection. The morbidity from this added procedure is slight. A similar attitude may be adopted for the submandibular gland. Radical neck dissections are not normally performed for malignant salivary gland tumours unless the neck involvement is massive.

In the case of minor salivary glands, it is usual to adopt a wait-and-see policy, responding surgically if the neck subsequently becomes involved.

Malignant tumours of salivary gland origin in children are excessively rare. They generally appear in the second decade, and roughly 50% are malignant with mucoepidermoid carcinomas predominating. It is wise to consider all childhood salivary gland tumours malignant until proven otherwise. However, preservation of the facial nerve is of paramount importance.

## Radiotherapy

Malignant salivary gland tumours are moderately radiosensitive, thus radiotherapy is employed in an adjunctive role, particularly when there are incomplete excision margins and when the tumour is high grade (Calman, 1995). Such combination therapy gives local control rates comparable with those when complete surgical clearance has been obtained.

Where the tumour is surgically unresectable, hyperfractionated radiotherapy to 70⁺Gy has been reported to give good control rates (Wang and Goodman, 1991), but there is no evidence of an improved survival benefit.

Fast neutron therapy has been advocated by Caterall and Errington (1987) as a means of treating unresectable malignant salivary gland tumours. However, the long-term morbidity of this treatment modality has now rendered it unacceptable according to RD Errington (personal communication, 1995).

# Outcome

A variety of factors play a role in the prognosis of patients with malignant salivary gland tumours. The chief factor is the grade of the tumour, with high-grade tumours having a worse prognosis. As with all malignant tumours, the degree of local development influences the outcome, with small tumours invariably having a better prognosis than large ones.

Carcinoma ex-pleomorphic adenoma and poorly differentiated adenocarcinomas fare least well, while the indolent nature of adenoid cystic carcinomas is well recognized. Unfortunately, the long-term survival of patients suffering from adenoid cystic carcinoma is poor, with few survivors at 20 years.

It is well recognized that patients with malignant tumours of the submandibular gland do less well than patients who have involvement of the parotid gland.

In the case of malignant minor salivary gland tumours, especially those of the oral cavity, there is an impression that survival is better than similar type tumours involving the major salivary glands. Unfortunately, it is difficult to confirm this impression, because of the rarity of these tumours.

# References

Ball ABS, Meirion Thomas J (1995) Malignant tumours of the major salivary glands. In: De Burgh Norman JE, McGurk M, eds. *Colour Atlas and Text of the Salivary Glands: Diseases, Disorders and Surgery*. Mosby Wolfe, London: 175

Bigger RJ, Curtis RE, Hoffman DA, Flannery JT (1983) Second primary malignancies following salivary gland cancer. *Br J Cancer* **46**: 383–6

Calman FMB (1995) Malignant tumours of the major salivary glands. In: De Burgh Norman JE, McGurk M, eds. *Colour Atlas and Text of the Salivary Glands: Diseases, Disorders and Surgery*. Mosby Wolfe, London: 190

Caterall M, Errington RD (1987) The implications of improved treatment of malignant salivary gland tumours by fast neutron radiotherapy. *Int J Radiat Oncol Biol Phys* **13**: 1313–18

Hollander L, Cunningham MP (1973) Management of cancer of the parotid gland. *Surg Clin N Am* **53**: 113

Jackson GL, Luna MA, Byers RM (1983) Results of surgery alone and surgery combined with postoperative radiotherapy in the treatment of cancer of the parotid gland. *Am J Surg* **146**: 497–500

Spiro RH (1986) Salivary neoplasms: overview of a 35-year experience with 2807 cases. *Head Neck Surg* **8**: 177–84

Vaughan ED, Richardson D (1993) Facial nerve reconstruction following ablative parotid surgery. *Br J Oral Maxillofac Surg* **5**: 274–80

Wang CC, Goodman M (1991) Photon irradiation of unresectable carcinomas of the salivary glands. *Int J Radiat Oncol Biol Phys* **21**: 569–76

Watkin GT, Hobsley M (1986) Influence of local surgery and radiotherapy on the natural history of pleomorphic adenomas. *Br J Surg* **73**: 74–6

# Chapter 11

# Diagnosis and management of thyroid eye disease

*Alastair Denniston, Paul Dodson, Tristan Reuser*

Recent advances are helping elucidate the pathogenesis and improve the management of thyroid eye disease. While biochemical investigations and imaging may be supportive, ophthalmological and medical clinical assessments remain the key to the diagnosis and management of this sight-threatening disorder.

Thyroid eye disease (TED) is an organ-specific autoimmune disorder, which may be both sight-threatening and disfiguring. Although clinical or biochemical thyroid dysfunction is present in most cases, it should be emphasized that, despite its name, patients with TED may be hyperthyroid, hypothyroid or euthyroid. Likewise, TED may precede, accompany or follow other evidence of thyroid dysfunction.

## Epidemiology

The annual incidence of TED is estimated at 16/100000 in females and 2.9/100000 in males (Bartley, 1994). It is commoner in middle age. The severe end of the spectrum tends to occur in older males, smokers and people with diabetes (with their associated microvascular disease), which is an important issue since the combination of diabetes and TED is not uncommon. Linked genes include human leukocyte antigen (HLA) DR3, HLA B8, cytotoxic lymphocyte-associated esterase-4 (CTLA4) and thyroid-stimulating hormone (TSH) receptor (Chistyakov et al, 2000).

## Pathology

Enlargement of extraocular muscles (EOM), fat and connective tissue occurs as a result of both the acute inflammation and an increase in glycosaminoglycans. Compression and inflammation of muscle fibres may result in fibrosis and atrophy in burnt-out disease. The cellular infiltrate consists of macrophages, T-cells, mast cells and occasional plasma cells (Bahn and Heufelder, 1993). Levels of T-cells (both CD4[+] and CD8[+]) and macrophages are much higher in early active disease (Pappa et al, 2000).

## Pathogenesis

Interestingly, the identity of both the target cell and the primary antigen remain in doubt. The fibroblast–adipocyte lineage are the strongest contenders based on early histological and cytochemical markers and the clinical parallels with pretibial myxoedema. The primary antigen probably shares epitopes with thyroid follicular cells; the TSH receptor remains one unproven candidate. Having escaped deletion by the immune system, recruitment of activated T-cells to the orbit is facilitated by cytokines (predominantly Th1 spectrum) and adhesion molecules (ICAM1, VCAM1, CD44) with subsequent clonal expansion. The ensuing barrage of cytokines, fibroblast growth factors and oxygen free radicals act upon the target cells to stimulate adipogenesis, fibroblast proliferation and glycosaminoglycan synthesis (Heufelder and Joba, 2000).

## Clinical features

TED is a clinical diagnosis. The cardinal features are lid retraction or lag (with characteristic visualization of sclera above the cornea), soft-tissue inflammation or infiltration, proptosis and restrictive myopathy of the extraocular muscles (Char, 1996).

### Lid retraction or lag

Retraction of the upper lid mainly results from shortening and tethering of the levator palpebrae superioris (LPS) (*Figure 11.1*). In addition, where there is tethering of the inferior rectus, further LPS elevation may arise from attempted corrective overaction of the superior rectus (neurologically part of the levator–superior rectus complex). Any proptosis will exacerbate the apparent lid retraction.

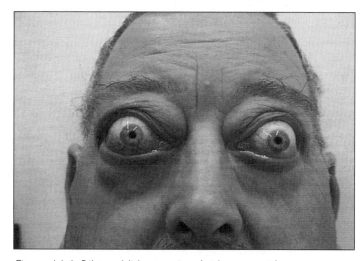

*Figure 11.1: Bilateral lid retraction (with proptosis).*

Lastly, overaction of the sympathetic part of the LPS (Muller's muscle) may occur as a result of thyroxine-induced sensitivity. Inferior lid retraction may also occur. When recording lid position, it should be remembered that the upper lid normally overlaps the superior limbus by 2 mm, whereas the lower lid rests on the inferior limbus.

### Soft-tissue signs

Common signs of active disease include conjunctival injection and oedema (chemosis), and oedema of the lids (*Figure 11.2*). Infiltration and forward prolapse of orbital fat may render the periorbital changes chronic. Inadequate lid closure as a result of proptosis may result in sight-threatening exposure keratopathy (*Figure 11.3*). This may be compounded by disease involvement of lacrimal glands and ensuing keratoconjunctivitis sicca.

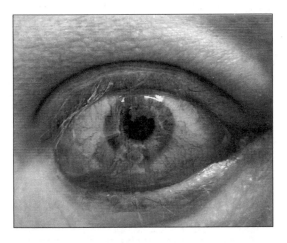

Figure 11.2: Chemosis, lid retraction and proptosis. This patient had a good response to orbital radiotherapy with steroid cover.

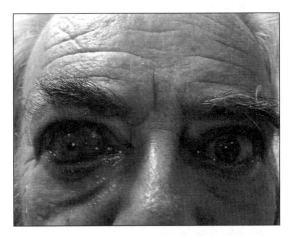

Figure 11.3: Diffuse fluorescein staining with hazy cornea indicative of exposure keratopathy in a proptotic right eye.

### Proptosis

TED is the commonest cause of proptosis (unilateral and bilateral) in adults (*Figures 11.1* and *11.2*). The adverse effect on vision at the front of the eye (exposure keratopathy) may be compounded by proptotic stretching of the optic nerve (contributing to optic neuropathy). This may actually be exacerbated by treatment because steroids may induce adipogenesis. It is easily measured with the Hertel's exophthalmometer.

## EOM enlargement/myopathy

Ocular motility may be disrupted by EOM changes. Initially, oedema and later fibrosis may restrict movement and cause diplopia. Interestingly, the rectus muscles tend to be affected in order: inferior, medial, superior and lastly lateral (*Figure 11.4*).

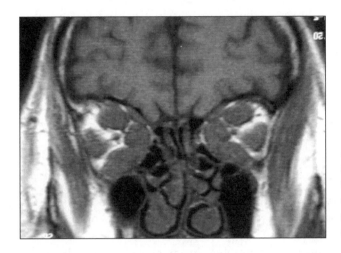

*Figure 11.4: Coronal magnetic resonance image showing the typical pattern of extraocular muscle involvement and compression of the optic nerve; the patient had minimal clinical signs other than ocular dysmotility.*

Involvement of the inferior rectus may be detected early by noting an increase in intraocular pressure on upward gaze. It should be noted that difficulties may occur in distinguishing inferior rectus restriction from a superior rectus palsy, or medial rectus restriction from a sixth nerve palsy, especially when there is little other evidence of TED.

## Optic neuropathy

Worsening visual acuity, altered colour perception and scotomata (blind spots) are important signs of optic nerve dysfunction, even though the optic disc commonly appears normal on ophthalmoscopy; in longstanding cases it may be atrophic, and vision will be irreversibly lost. Colour vision may be usefully monitored with Ishihara pseudoisochromatic plates or by comparing colour intensity of a stimulus with both eyes. The neuropathy may be caused by stretch or compression by the surrounding swollen recti muscles (*Figure 11.4*).

## Systemic associations

It is important that a full medical examination is carried out to assess thyroid status, thyroid gland abnormalities, such as a goitre, and systemic features, such as pretibial myxoedema and thyroid acropachy.

# Investigation

### Thyroid function tests

TSH (released from the pituitary) and free thyroxine measurement are the most commonly measured indices of thyroid function. However, if these are normal yet clinical suspicion remains, free tri-iodothyronine (the more active metabolite) should be measured. TSH is commonly suppressed in TED and may be an early marker of thyroid disease. Antithyroglobulin, antiperoxidase and TSH receptor antibodies are commonly associated with TED.

### Imaging

Orbital imaging is important for diagnosis and to plan management.

Computed tomography (CT) has been largely superseded by magnetic resonance imaging (MRI), although CT bony windows may still have a role in planning decompression operations (Trokel and Jacobiec, 1981).

MRI avoids ionizing radiation, permits image reconstruction in any plane and provides much better soft tissue detail, allowing assessment of disease activity and any impending optic neuropathy (Kahaly et al, 1995).

# Management

### General

In managing TED, the following should be considered:

⌘ assessment (*Figure 11.5)*
⌘ counselling
⌘ symptomatic measures
⌘ medical options for active disease
⌘ surgical options (mainly for inactive disease).

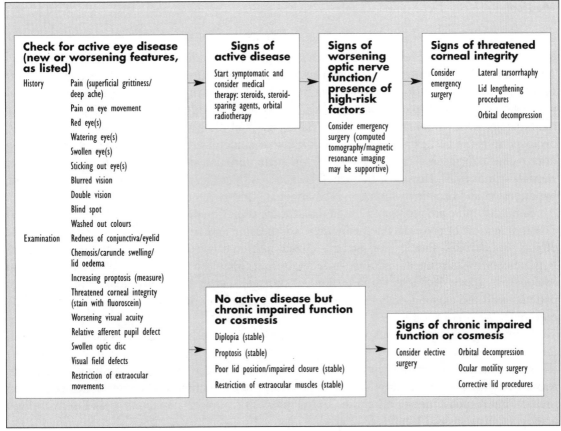

*Figure 11.5: Ophthalmic assessment of the patient with thyroid eye disease.*

The presence of poor prognostic features may guide towards a more aggressive therapeutic approach (*Table 11.1*).

Multidisciplinary input may be effectively delivered by a combined clinic comprising both endocrine and ophthalmic services. Thus, the aims of euthyroidism and control of eye disease may be coordinated. Counselling should include the reassurance that TED is a self-limiting disease. Local and national support groups are often helpful.

Symptomatic measures include ocular lubricants, tinted glasses, bed-head elevation (to combat morning exacerbation of symptoms) and prisms for diplopia.

### Table 11.1: High-risk group

The following are risk factors for a worse final outcome and may require a more aggressive approach:

Older age of onset

Male

Smoker

Diabetes

Reduced visual acuity

Rapid progression at onset

Length of disease

## Medical

In the active stage, the severe forms of disease are generally predicted by a more aggressive onset. These patients therefore require frequent review and careful documentation of ocular and optic nerve function. This is also the group most likely to benefit from medical immunosuppression — with steroids, steroid-sparing agents (e.g. cyclosporin, methotrexate, azathioprine), orbital radiotherapy or a combination of these (Bartalena et al, 2000). Of the steroid-sparing agents, cyclosporin is the best established, with prospective randomized, controlled trials demonstrating improvement in disease control (when given with steroids) and a reduced relapse rate (after steroids withdrawal). However, the benefit was offset by frequent side effects, notably infection, hypertension and hepatic dysfunction (Kahaly et al, 1986).

Similarly, there are promising initial data for the use of methotrexate, but close monitoring is essential in view of potential haematopoietic suppression and hepatic toxicity. However, the side effects of steroids should not be trivialized and may also require monitoring, such as hypertension, gastrointestinal side effects (which may be treated prophylactically) and osteoporosis (bone densitometry in prolonged courses). Furthermore, glycaemic control both in patients with pre-existing diabetes and to pick up those who develop diabetes *de novo* is also required.

Immunosuppression by radiotherapy appears to be as effective as steroids with, so far, minimal side effects (Prummel et al, 1993; Mourits et al, 2000). The transient exacerbation of disease severity associated with radiotherapy may be reduced by simultaneous steroid administration, and this is now standard practice. Other immunomodulators under evaluation include intravenous immunoglobulin, plasmapharesis, cytokine antagonists and somatostatin analogues (Krassas and Heufelder, 2001).

There has been widespread debate over the activation or worsening of TED as a result of antithyroid treatments. While this is most marked with the use of radioiodine-131 ([131]I), it is also seen in association with thyroidectomy and medical antithyroid therapy; it is postulated that this occurs as a result of autoimmune activation to thyroid antigens in the context of thyroid injury. Significantly, the largest randomized study of [131]I and its effects on TED demonstrated that the rate of activation or worsening of TED associated with [131]I was abolished if steroids were given simultaneously (15% *vs* 0%) (Bartalena et al, 1998); however, this study only included patients with mild or no evidence of TED and was not controlled for other risk factors (e.g. smoking, diabetes). Thyroidectomy appears to have a less dramatic effect on activation or worsening of TED, and there is probably no additional benefit from steroids; debate continues as to whether subtotal thyroidectomy has a relatively worse effect on TED compared with total thyroidectomy (reviewed by Bartalena et al, 2000).

## Surgical

Where medical treatment proves inadequate, optic nerve compression and severe corneal involvement are indications for emergency orbital decompression. Decompression options include the extent (two-, three- or four-wall) and approach (transorbital, transantral or endoscopic). Most commonly, the two-wall (floor and medial wall) decompression is used (*Figures 11.6* and *11.7*). If the cornea is threatened but there is no danger of optic nerve compression, a temporary lateral or central tarsorrhaphy may be sufficient.

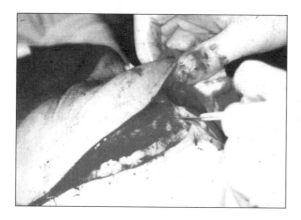

*Figure 11.6: Coronal approach to decompression; incision relatively hidden by the hairline.*

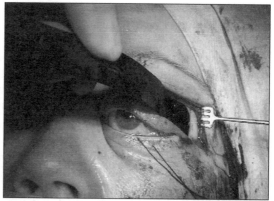

*Figure 11.7: Anterior approach to decompression; incision relatively hidden by a skin crease.*

In burnt-out or inactive disease, surgery may permit restoration of normal vision and cosmesis (*Figures 11.8* and *11.9*).

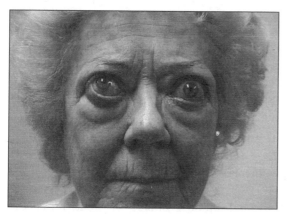

*Figure 11.8: 'Burnt out' thyroid eye disease with proptosis, lid retraction and ocular dysmotility.*

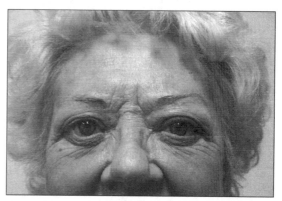

*Figure 11.9: The same patient shortly after orbital decompression. In some cases, ocular dysmotility resolves with decompression alone.*

The psychological effects of the changed appearance should not be underestimated. Patients have been known to go into 'voluntary' social isolation because of the perceived frightful appearance (Gerding et al, 1997).

Surgical options comprise orbital decompression, motility surgery and lid procedures:

⌘ Orbital decompression deals with proptosis, which may be both disfiguring and threaten corneal and optic nerve integrity

⌘ Motility surgery to regain binocular single vision usually involves recession of the medial and/or inferior rectus, with adjustable sutures. This should only be attempted when motility has been stable for 6 months

⌘ Lid operations may improve corneal protection and/or cosmesis by reducing lower lid retraction (recession of lower lid retractors), upper lid retraction (release of levator aponeurosis, excision of Muller's muscle) or both (lateral tarsorrhaphy).

Redundant skin and fatty tissues may be removed by blepharoplasty; laser techniques also have an emerging role by making the procedure virtually bloodless.

## Conclusion

TED is a familiar condition but which has, as yet, no clear cause (the target cell and antigen remain uncertain), no confirmatory test and no specific cure. It may well be that the discovery of the first will lead to both an accurate diagnostic test and a targeted cure. For now, clinical assessment remains the key to both diagnosis and treatment selection. According to disease severity and activity, both immunomodulation and surgery have a role in combating this sight-threatening and disfiguring disease.

## References

Bahn RS, Heufelder AE (1993) Pathogenesis of Graves' ophthalmopathy. *N Engl J Med* **329**: 1468–75

Bartalena L, Marcocci C, Bogazzi F et al (1998) Relation between therapy for hyperthyroidism and the course of Graves' ophthalmopathy. *N Engl J Med* **338**: 73–8

Bartalena L, Pinchera A, Marcocci C (2000) Management of Graves' ophthalmopathy: reality and perspectives. *Endocr Rev* **21**: 168–99

Bartley GB (1994) Epidemiologic characteristics and clinical course of ophthalmopathy associated with autoimmune thyroid disease in Olmstead County, Minnesota. *Trans Am Ophthalmol Soc* **92**: 477–588

Char DH (1996) Thyroid eye disease. *Br J Ophthalmol* **80**: 922–6

Chistyakov DA, Savost'anov KV, Turakulov RI, Nosikov VV (2000) Genetic determinants of Graves disease. *Mol Genet Metab* **71**(1-2): 66–9

Gerding MN, Terwee CB, Dekker FW, Koornneef L, Prummel MF, Wiersinga WM (1997) Quality of life in patients with Graves' ophthalmopathy is markedly decreased: measurement by the Medical Outcomes Study Instrument. *Thyroid* **7**: 885–9

Heufelder AE, Joba W (2000) Thyroid-associated eye disease. *Strabismus* **8**(2): 101–11

Kahaly G, Schrezenmeir J, Krause U, Schweikert B, Meuer S, Muller W (1986) Ciclosporin and prednisone *vs* prednisone in treatment of Graves' ophthalmopathy: a controlled, randomized and prospective study. *Eur J Clin Invest* **16**: 415–22

Kahaly G, Diaz M, Just M, Beyer J, Lieb W (1995) Role of octreoscan and correlation with MR imaging in Graves' ophthalmopathy. *Thyroid* **5**(2): 107–11

Krassas GE, Heufelder AE (2001) Immunosuppressive therapy in patients with thyroid eye disease: an overview of current concepts. *Eur J Endocrinol* **144**(4): 311–18

Mourits MP, Kempen van-Harteveld L, Garcia MB, Koppeschaar HP, Tick L, Terwee CB (2000) Radiotherapy for Graves' orbitopathy: randomised, placebo-controlled study. *Lancet* **355**: 1505–9

Pappa A, Lawson JM, Calder V, Fells P, Lightman S (2000) T cells and fibroblasts in early and late thyroid associated ophthalmopathy. *Br J Ophthalmol* **84**(5): 517–22

Prummel MF, Mourits MP, Blank L, Koornneef L, Wiersinga WM (1993) Randomised double blind trial of prednisone vs radiotherapy in Graves' ophthalmopathy. *Lancet* **342**: 949–54

Trokel SL, Jacobiec FA (1981) Correlation of CT scanning and pathological features of ophthalmic Graves' disease. *Ophthalmology* **88**(6): 553–64

# Chapter 12

# Snoring: recent developments

*TM Jones, Andrew C Swift*

Despite limited evidence validating its efficacy, surgery to overcome snoring is commonly undertaken. This chapter looks at the development of snoring surgery to present day, highlighting its limitations and outlining current methods being used to target the surgery more effectively.

Snoring is a common malady (Fairbanks and Fujita, 1987). Estimates of prevalence of habitual snoring ranges from 24–50% for men (Katsantonis et al, 1988; Woodhead et al, 1991; Maniglia, 1993) and from 14–30% for women (Fairbanks and Fujita, 1987; Ah-See et al, 1998).

Snoring noise, or stertorous sleep-related breathing, is generated by the vibration of anatomical structures of the upper aerodigestive tract during sleep, combined with the sound of turbulent airflow. Sleep results in a muscular hypotonia and consequent segmental collapse of oropharyngeal and/or hypopharyngeal structures. This collapse is exacerbated, according to the Bernoulli phenomenon, by the negative intraluminal pressure created by inspiratory airflow (Gavriely and Jensen, 1993); the net effect is obstruction of the supraglottic airway. An inspiratory effort has to be generated to overcome this airway collapse. If the collapse results in complete airway closure and the forces contributing to the collapse exceed an undefined critical threshold, an apnoeic episode usually results, and arousal is required to generate an adequate voluntary inspiratory effort to overcome the collapse. If, however, the collapse is partial, or the contributing forces do not exceed threshold, a greater inspiratory effort, generated involuntarily during sleep without arousal, will be sufficient to overcome the collapse. In either case the enhanced respiratory effort will result in a greater airflow velocity.

Potential contributors to the generation of snoring sound include the vibration of upstream structures (e.g. soft palate), vibrating oscillations of the airway walls at the point of maximal collapse as well as the turbulent nature of airflow itself (Beck et al, 1995). Which structure actually vibrates depends on many factors, few of which are well understood (Perez-Padilla et al, 1993). In most cases, the soft palate is assumed to be the primary noise generator, although other structures of the supraglottis or oropharynx, as well as tongue base and epiglottis, may also vibrate to a greater or lesser extent in any one individual (Quinn et al, 1995).

Snoring is a symptom of sleep–related breathing dysfunction, which is usually considered as a continuum, with 'uncomplicated' snoring at one extreme and obstructive sleep apnoea syndrome (OSAS) at the other (Lugaresi et al, 1978; Issa and Sullivan, 1984). Snoring is worse in men than in women, and is known to worsen with age, obesity, alcohol ingestion and nasal obstruction (Fairbanks, 1990; Stradling and Crosby, 1991).

In its simplest form, snoring results in considerable social disability, contributing to relationship disharmony, marriage breakdown, social ostrasization and even murder (Edilberto et al, 1989). In addition, apparent uncomplicated snoring has been identified as a contributory factor towards hypertension, ischaemic heart disease and cerebrovascular accident, as well as increased morbidity and mortality from road traffic and work-related accidents (Koskenvuo et al, 1985; Partinen and Palomaki, 1985; Koskenvuo et al, 1987; Haraldsson et al, 1995).

OSAS is a serious medical condition, which if not treated may result in physical and/or psychological morbidity or even death (Guilleminault et al, 1976; Tilkian et al, 1977; Clark, 1979; Kales et al, 1985; Hung et al, 1990; Bédard et al, 1991; Fletcher, 1995). It is not sufficient to treat OSAS sufferers as snorers (Krespi et al, 1994). With this in mind, although surgery has been used to treat OSAS, we will not consider it further in this chapter. It is most common for physicians with an interest in sleep medicine to treat OSAS sufferers with a nasal continuous positive airway pressure appliance (Wright and Dye, 1995).

## Assessment of snorers

Snorers are typically referred to otolaryngologists or respiratory physicians with an interest in snoring and sleep-related breathing disorders.

On initial assessment, particular care is taken to elicit evidence of any medical complications of OSAS. Depending on the history and examination findings, one of several screening procedures may be invoked. For individuals with a low index of suspicion of OSAS, an overnight pulse oximetry will suffice. However, if the index of suspicion is high, a formal polysomnography is perfomed.

Nasal obstruction, collar size, body mass index and alcohol and cigarette consumption are also documented as they have all been implicated in snoring severity (Stradling and Crosby, 1991; Hoijer et al, 1992; Braver et al, 1995; Koay et al, 1995; Wenzel et al, 1997; Ah-See et al, 1998).

## Treatment of simple snorers

### *Conservative*

Surgery is not the only means by which reduction of snoring may be achieved. Several conservative methods have been shown to be effective, such as weight reduction, reduction of alcohol intake and treatment of coincident nasal obstruction (Stradling and Crosby, 1991; Hoijer et al, 1992; Braver et al, 1995; Wenzel et al, 1997).

Attendance to these may have significant effects on the reduction of snoring and should be attempted before consideration of any surgical remedy. It should be emphasised that if any of these factors remain untreated, the chances of surgical success is likely to be compromised.

Mandibular advancement prostheses (*Figure 12.1a,b*) are used to reduce snoring and improve OSAS (Schmidt-Nowara et al, 1995; Stradling et al, 1998). They consist of an upper and lower dental bite-plate fixed together. The mechanics are such that when the bite-plates are in position on the upper and lower teeth, the force transmitted from one to the other promotes protrusion of the mandible. They are used during sleep and serve to pull the tongue forward, resulting in an increased oro- and hypopharyngeal diameter, thereby relieving airway collapse, which is the underlying cause of the snoring. Recent work has shown that approximately 55% of patients are able to tolerate long-term use. Of these, 97% considered them effective in reducing snoring (McGown et al, 2001).

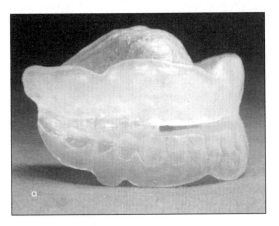 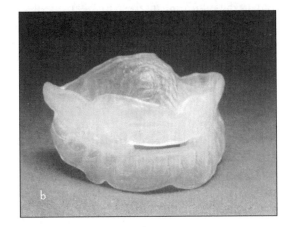

Figure 12.1a,b: Mandibular advancement prostheses.

## Surgical

### Uvulopalatopharyngoplasty

Uvulopalatopharyngoplasty (UPPP) (*Figure 12.2a,b,c*) was pioneered in 1964 by Ikematsu and introduced to the West by Fujita et al in 1981 as a surgical remedy for OSAS. The procedure includes a tonsillectomy, or de-epithelialization of the tonsillar fossae if tonsillectomy has already been performed, followed by suture apposition of the denuded anterior and posterior faucal pillars, followed by excision of 1–2 cm of the soft palate including the uvula.

Use of the technique to cure uncomplicated snoring increased over the subsequent decade. Although it has been shown to reduce snoring, results were variable (Blair Simmonds et al, 1984; Sharp et al, 1990; Koay et al, 1995). Moreover, it became apparent with time that there were significant and unacceptable complications. These included nasal regurgitation, nasopharyngeal stenosis, hypernasal voice and even death (Croft and Golding-Wood, 1990; Fairbanks, 1990).

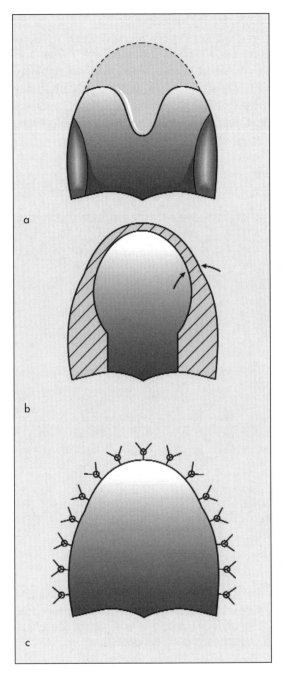

*Figure 12.2. Uvulopalatopharyngoplasty. a and b. Tonsillectomy and excision of uvula and rim of soft palate. c. Apposition of mucosal edges.*

## Palatoplasty procedures

In an attempt to overcome the radical nature of UPPP, its complications and uncertain outcome, a variety of techniques that were limited to the soft palate were devised. These are all based on the supposition that palatal flutter is one of the most important sound generator mechanisms of snore production. Therefore, reducing palatal flutter or vibration should, in theory, reduce the level of snoring. These techniques are based on one of two themes:

⌘ either to reduce the length of the soft palate *and/or*

⌘ to stiffen the soft palate.

## Palatal stiffening techniques

In the early 1990s, Ellis et al proposed a radical change in strategy for the treatment of uncomplicated snoring by the introduction of palatal stiffening.

His technique used a laser to remove a central longitudinal strip of mucosa from the oral surface of the soft palate and uvula. Subsequent healing by fibrosis resulted in the required stiffening of the soft palate and, at least in the short term, a reduction of snoring noise (Ellis et al, 1993; Ellis, 1994).

Several different techniques have been developed since. These include:

⌘ diathermy-assisted uvulopalatoplasty (DAUP) (Yardley et al, 1997)

⌘ laser palatoplasty plus excision of the uvula (Morar et al, 1995; Ingrams et al, 1996) (*Figure 12.3a,b*)

⌘ simple soft palate cautery (Mair and Day, 1996).

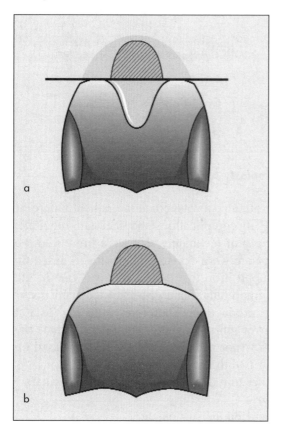

*Figure 12.3. Palatoplasty plus uvulectomy. a. Mucosal flap excised from soft palate. b. Uvulectomy.*

This technique involves sequential removal of soft palate lateral to the base of the uvula, resulting in the formation of bilateral 'Kamami trenches'. Formation of the trenches leads to a relative elongation of the uvula, which, though spared, is shortened as the trenches are elongated. In order to prevent excess removal of palatal tissue and to allow assessment of effectiveness, patients were required to undergo several procedures, separated by a 4–6-week interval, with only a small strip of palate vapourized at each visit.

## Palatal shortening techniques

*Laser-assisted uvulopalatoplasty.* Kamami (1990) described laser-assisted uvulopalatoplasty (LAUP) (*Figure 12.4a,b*), and the procedure has been widely used since (Carenfelt, 1991; Krespi and Pearlman, 1995; Wareing and Mitchell, 1996; Ikeda et al, 1997).

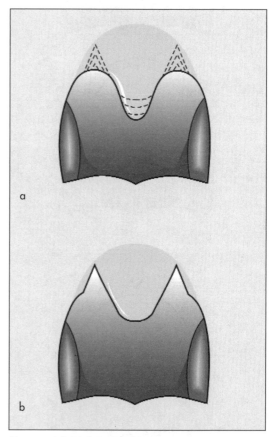

*Figure 12.4: Laser-assisted uvulopalatoplasty. a. Sequential excision of soft palate 'trenches'. b. Sequential shortening of uvula.*

Each procedure was carried out using local anaesthesia in the 'office' setting. Kamami reported a success rate comparable with UPPP, with a marked decrease in postoperative complications. He did concede, however, that the requirement for repeated procedures was a significant drawback to the technique.

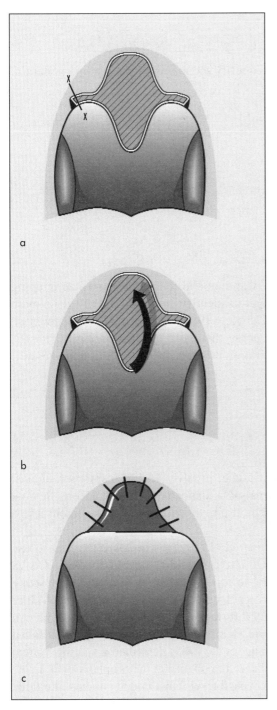

*Figure 12.5. Flap palatoplasty. a. Lateral releasing incisions (X–X), and mucosal strip from soft palate and uvula. b. Uvula flap anteverted onto soft palate. c. Flap secured with vicryl.*

*Uvulopalatal elevation palatoplasty.* In this technique, a laser is used to excise a mucosal strip from the oral surface of the soft palate and uvula (*Figure 12.5a,b,c*).

Lateral palatal incisions release the soft palate, allowing the uvula flap to be reflected anteriorly onto the denuded oral surface of the soft palate. It is secured with vicryl sutures. Covering the raw area of the soft palate has been shown to minimize postoperative pain and discomfort (Wilde and Swift, 1995).

Whichever technique is used, palatoplasty surgery confers several advantages over UPPP (Kamami, 1990; Ellis et al, 1993; Krespi and Pearlman, 1995; Morar et al, 1995; Ingrams et al, 1996; Mair and Day, 1996; Clarke et al, 1998):

⌘ The results are good, at least in the short term
⌘ There is minimal voice change
⌘ The incidence of nasal regurgitation and nasopharyngeal stenosis is also decreased.

Palatoplasty surgery does, however, appear to result in significant early postoperative pain (Clarke et al, 1998), and there is an attendant initial failure rate of 7–22% (Ikeda et al, 1997).

Primary failure of the procedure probably occurs because palatal flutter may not be the major mechanism of sound production in every individual. Therefore, negating palatal flutter in such individuals is unlikely to remedy their snoring.

Considerable effort has been applied in an attempt to target palatal procedures more precisely, avoiding unnecessary surgery in up to 25% of snorers seeking help.

# Targeting palatal surgery

Several techniques have been used in an attempt to identify the major snoring sound generator mechanism in any one individual. These include:

- imaging
- the Müller Manoeuvre
- sedation (sleep) nasendoscopy
- acoustic analysis.

## *Imaging*

Fluoroscopic techniques, computerized tomography, scanning and magnetic resonance imaging (both static and dynamic) have been used in attempts to identify structures involved in snore generation with only limited success (Shepard and Thawley, 1989; Ryan et al, 1991; Jäger et al, 1998). Practicability and excess radiation exposure prove the major limitations. Consequently, these techniques have found no place in the preoperative assessment of the non-apnoeic anti-social snorer.

## *The Müller Manoeuvre*

The Müller Manoeuvre, performed in the outpatient clinic, involves forced inspiration against closed nasal and oral airways (i.e. the opposite of a valsalva manoeuvre). Simultaneous flexible nasendoscopy enables direct visualization of the extent of airway collapse at the different levels during the Manoeuvre.

Its use developed from the early work of Weitzman et al (1978), who were the first to use fibreoptic endoscopy (albeit in patients who were asleep) to assess pharyngeal collapse in OSAS sufferers. Borowiecki and Sassin (1983) were the first to report the use of fibreoptic endoscopy in awake patients, demonstrating generalized pharyngeal collapse on performing the Müller Manoeuvre. Sher et al (1986) developed the technique further, showing differential segmental collapse of the pharynx during the Müller Manoeuvre in a group of patients with craniofacial anomalies who suffered OSAS. In a separate paper, Sher et al (1985) described a scoring system based on the extent of collapse at the velopharynx relative to collapse at the oropharyngeal level. From the comparative scores of the extent of collapse at each level they divided patients into three groups: 'ideal', 'suboptimal but acceptable' and 'unsuitable'. Separation of patients into each group allowed prediction of surgical success.

However, the technique has subsequently been shown to be inferior to other techniques, such as sleep nasendoscopy (Pringle and Croft, 1991). Furthermore, recent work, using specific acoustic parameters of snoring sound as objective outcome measurements of palatal surgery, showed the Müller Manoeuvre to have a specificity of 55.5% and a sensitivity of 30.4% in predicting surgical success (Jones, 2005). Few surgeons still consider the Müller Manoeuvre to be of value in the preoperative assessment of snorers, and therefore it is now rarely used to select individuals for snoring surgery (Boot et al, 1997).

### Sedation (sleep) nasendoscopy

Sedation (sleep) nasendoscopy was first described by Croft and Pringle in 1991 and later simplified by Camilleri et al in 1995, and requires the patient to be sedated. Once snoring is achieved, a nasendoscope is used in an attempt to visualize the vibrating structures contributing to the snoring sound. It would be expected that only patients in whom soft palate flutter dominates would benefit from a palatoplasty procedure. However, the technique has two major flaws:

⌘ First, it is unlikely that sedation-induced sleep correlates well with natural sleep. Therefore, the respective mechanisms of snoring may have little in common
⌘ Second, there is currently no standardized protocol for sedation. This results in wide variation from individual to individual, between sequential studies on the same individual and between centres (Camilleri et al, 1995; Quinn et al, 1995; Marais, 1998; Takeda, 1998).

It has again recently been shown, using specific acoustic parameters of snoring sound as objective outcome measurements of palatal surgery, that a sensitivity of 50.0% and a specificity of 62.5% is possible if the Croft and Pringle grading system is employed, compared with a sensitivity of 90.9% and a specificity of 33.3% for the Camilleri system (Jones, 2005). Moreover, comparison of the acoustics of natural snoring with snores induced at increasing levels of sedation show significant differences. These differences were highly significant, even at the lowest sedation levels that snoring was induced, providing further evidence that a different mechanism of snore production between natural and sedation-induced snores is likely (Jones, 2005). Other studies using subjective outcome data concur with these findings (El Badawey et al, 2003).

Therefore, as with the Müller Manoeuvre, sleep nasendoscopic findings, scored using these classifications, cannot be recommended as a reliable predictor of the outcome of palatal surgery in non-apnoeic snorers.

### Acoustic analysis

Since the early 1990s, interest in the acoustic analysis of the snoring sound has developed. Acoustic techniques have been used in an effort to create theoretical models of snoring sound production (Gavriely and Jensen, 1993; Beck et al, 1995). Additionally, snoring sound has been used to diagnose OSAS (Perez-Padilla et al, 1993; McCombe et al, 1995; Fiz et al, 1996), as an objective outcome measurement of snoring surgery (Prichard et al, 1995; Smithson et al, 1995; Walker et al, 1996) and in an attempt to differentiate the underlying mechanism of sound generation (Weingarten and Raviv, 1995).

In order to predict the outcome of palatal surgery acoustically, the specific acoustic characteristics of palatal flutter would have to be determined.

Several groups have employed the technique of sleep nasendoscopy while simultaneously recording snores produced, in an attempt to identify acoustic parameters specific to palatal flutter (Quinn et al, 1996; Agarwal et al, 2002; Osborne et al, 1999). They hoped that screening of natural snoring sound for relative composition of sound generated by palatal flutter would then allow individual patient selection for surgical intervention. In each case, they demonstrated that snoring resulting from palatal flutter was of a lower frequency than snoring sound generated by other mechanisms.

Osborne et al (1999) observed that the digital soundwave of snoring sound, known to be caused by palatal flutter (as seen on sleep nasendoscopic examination), contained regular explosive peaks of sound occurring at approximately 20 Hz frequency. Such peaks were not seen when the snoring sound was generated by non-palatal vibration. In order to quantify these differences between palatal and non-palatal snores, they calculated the ratio of peak sound amplitude (99th centile) to the root mean square (RMS) amplitude (effective average sound amplitude) for each 0.2 second segment of the snoring sound (*Figure 12.6*). They postulated, and subsequently demonstrated, that the greater the contribution of palatal futter to the overall snoring sound, the higher the numerical value of the ratio.

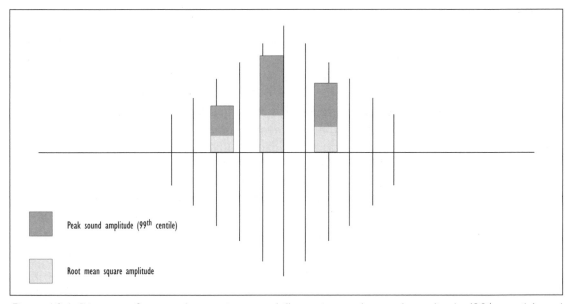

Peak sound amplitude (99th centile)

Root mean square amplitude

*Figure 12.6: Diagram of a complex snoring sound illustrating peak sound amplitude (99th centile) and root mean square amplitude of three 0.2 second divisions.*

Following the investigation of 11 non-apnoeic snorers, they were able to show that a peak to RMS ratio >2.70 was characteristic of palatal snores, while values <2.70 were characteristic of lower segment snores, and that this may allow selection of patients for palatal surgery. However, when the peak to RMS ratio was assessed in light of objective, acoustic outcomes of snoring surgery, prediction of surgical outcome was not possible (Jones, 2005).

An additional acoustic parameter designed to identify the palatal component of a snore is the simulated snore (SS) ratio. Its derivation followed observations that simulated snoring sound in an awake individual is generated predominantly by palatal flutter. It was proposed that, if simulated snoring sound is 'subtracted' from natural snoring sound, for any given individual, the residual sound will constitute the non-palatal sound element of the natural snore. The SS ratio is the ratio of the average energy of a natural snore to the average residual energy after the simulated snoring sound has been subtracted. This is calculated using the signal processing techniques inverse filtration and linear prediction analysis. Linear prediction analysis allows calculation of the contribution of the simulated snoring sound to the overall natural snoring sound. Subsequent inverse filtration enables calculation of the residual difference between the two.

The smaller the residual, the greater the per cent of palatal flutter in the 'natural' snore and the bigger the numerical value of the SS ratio. Therefore, the bigger the SS ratio, the more successful the expected outcome from palatal surgery. However, as with the peak to RMS ratio, when the SS ratio was assessed in light of objective, acoustic outcomes of snoring surgery, prediction of surgical outcome was not possible (Jones, 2005).

## Long-term outcome

Another recent study that used a specifically designed questionnaire to assess snoring outcome provides a longer postoperative follow-up than any other study published. It shows that of a cohort of 193 patients who underwent surgery for snoring, 23.7% reported no improvement at all in their snoring postoperatively, 42.7% reported an initial improvement that was not sustained for 2 years, while 33.6% reported an improvement that was sustained for at least 2 years (Jones et al, 2005a).

These results are similar to those of a recent, randomized controlled trial in which specific acoustic parameters of snoring sound were used to assess outcome. In this trial, 42% of patients undergoing palatal surgery for snoring derived no acoustic benefit from surgery, while 58% had an initial benefit. However, only 38% had sustained benefit at follow-up between 5.9–17.5 months postoperatively (Jones et al, 2005b).

## New developments

The great demand for treatment by patients who snore loudly has lead to the development of alternative interventional therapies that are widely advertised by the media and the internet. These techniques rely on being quick and easy for the patient to undergo in an 'office' setting using local anaesthesia, thus avoiding hospital admission. They are generally less painful than surgical palatoplasty, are minimally invasive and have low morbidity with few complications. However, several treatments may be required to induce an improvement in snoring.

The techniques include:

- *Somnoplasty*™. This is a technique of delivering controlled-radiofrequency thermal abalation (RFA) to the soft palate. This heats the tissue to 60–90°C, inducing a limited lesion that will later form a scar and stiffen the soft palate
- *Bipolar radiofrequency-induced thermotherapy (RFITT)*. The Celon method is similar to Somnoplasty™, but the technique uses automatic dosimetry and an acoustic feedback signal
- *Coblation*™. This technique uses radiofrequency technology and saline delivered by a wand to dissolve and remove tissue from the soft palate and induce scarring
- *Injection snoreplasty*. The soft palate is injected with a sclerosant such as alcohol, sodium tetradecyl sulphate or collagen to induce fibrosis and palatal stiffening
- *Palatal implants*. Braided polyethylene terephthalate (PET) is implanted into the soft palate and subsequently causes fibrosis.

The radiofrequency methods can also be used on additional structures such as the inferior turbinates, tonsils and tongue base to try and control snoring.

Subjective data suggest that the above treatment modalities are effective but this has not been confirmed by objective studies; there is a great need for careful audit and research into their long-term effects before any firm conclusions can be made.

## Conclusion

Surgery to alleviate antisocial snoring is still commonly performed in the UK, with over 11 000 patients undergoing a surgical procedure each year (Department of Health, 1996). This adds a significant financial burden on the health service budget.

A recent systematic review has confirmed that few of the techniques currently used have undergone rigorous evaluation. Of the prospective trials that exist, few are randomized correctly, and even those that are rely on subjective data (Jones and Ah-See, 2005).

In summary, only approximately one-third of patients who undergo snoring surgery achieve sustained benefit; thus approximately two-thirds enjoy only a temporary improvement at best. Despite considerable effort, it is not possible at present to predict the third of patients who appear to enjoy sustained benefit. Therefore, future research directed towards the development of strategies to reliably target these individuals preoperatively would seem advisable.

## References

Agarwal S, Stone P, McGuiness K, Morris J, Camilleri AE (2002) Sound frequency analysis and the site of snoring in natural and sedation-induced sleep. *Clin Otolaryngol* **27**(3): 162–6

Ah-See KW, Banham SW, Carter R, Stewart M, Robinson K, Wilson JA (1998) Systematic analysis of snoring in women. *Ann Otol Rhinol Laryngol* **107**: 227–31

Bédard MA, Montplaisir J, Richer F, Rouleau I, Malo J (1991) Obstructive sleep apnea syndrome: pathogenesis of neuropsychological deficits. *J Clin Exp Neuropsychol* **113**(6): 950–64

Beck R, Odeh M, Oliven A, Gravriely N (1995) The acoustic properties of snores. *Eur Respir J* **8**: 2120–8

Blair Simmonds F, Guilleminault C, Miles LE (1984) The palatopharyngoplasty operation for snoring and sleep apnoea: an interim report. *Otolaryngol Head Neck Surg* **92**: 375–80

Boot H, Poublon RML, Van Wegen R et al (1997) Uvulopalatopharyngoplasty for the obstructive sleep apnoea syndrome: value of polysomnography, Müller manoeuvre and cephalometry in predicting surgical outcome. *Clin Otolaryngol* **22**: 504–10

Borowiecki B, Sassin J (1983) Surgical treatment of sleep apnoea. *Arch Otolaryngol* **109**: 508

Braver HM, Block AJ, Perri MG (1995) Treatment for snoring. Combined weight loss, sleeping on side and nasal spray. *Chest* **107**(5): 1283–8

Camilleri AE, Ramamurthy L, Jones PH (1995) Sleep nasendoscopy: what benefit to the management of snorers? *J Laryngol Otol* **109**: 1163–5

Carenfelt C (1991) Laser uvulopalatoplasty in treatment of habitual snoring. *Ann Otol Rhinol Laryngol* **100**: 451–4

Clark RW (1979) Sleep apnea. *Primary Care* **6**: 653–79

Clarke RW, Yardley MPJ, Davies CM, Panarese A, Clegg RT, Parker AJ (1998) Palatoplasty for snoring: a randomised controlled trial of three surgical methods. *Otolaryngol Head Neck Surg* **119**: 288–92

Croft CB, Golding-Wood DG (1990) Uses and complications of uvulopalatopharyngoplasty. *J Laryngol Otol* **104**: 871–5

Croft CB, Pringle M (1991) Sleep nasendoscopy: a technique of assessment in snoring and obstructive sleep apnoea. *Clin Otolaryngol* **16**: 504–9

Department of Health (1995) *Hospital Episode Statistics*. DoH, London

Edilberto MAJ, Pelausa O, Tarshis LM (1989) Surgery for snoring. *Laryngoscope* **99**: 1006–10

El Badawey MR, McKee G, Heggie N, Marshall H, Wilson JA (2003) Predictive value of sleep nasendoscopy in the management of habitual snorers. *Ann Otol Rhinol Laryngol* **112**: 40–4

Ellis PDM (1994) Laser palatoplasty for snoring due to palatal flutter: a further report. *Clin Otolaryngol* **19**: 350–1

Ellis PDM, Ffowcs Williams JE, Shneerson JM (1993) Surgical relief of snoring due to palatal flutter: a preliminary report. *Ann R Coll Surg Engl* **75**: 286–290

Fairbanks DNF (1990) UVPP complications and avoidance strategies. *Otolaryngol Head Neck Surg* **102**: 239–45

Fairbanks DNF, Fujita S (1987) *Snoring and Obstructive Sleep Apnea*. Raven Press, New York: 1–18

Fiz JA, Abad J, Jané R et al (1996) Acoustic analysis of snoring sound in patients with simple snoring and obstructive sleep apnoea. *Eur Respir J* **9**: 2365–70

Fletcher EC (1995) The relationship between systemic hypertension and obstructive sleep apnea: facts and theory. *Am J Med* **98**: 118–28

Fujita S, Conway W, Zorick F, Roth T (1981) Surgical correction of anatomic abnormalities in obstructive sleep apnea syndrome: uvulopalatopharyngoplasty. *Otolaryngol Head Neck Surg* **89**: 923–34

Gavriely N, Jensen O (1993) Theory and measurement of snores. *J Appl Physiol* **74**(6): 2828–37

Guilleminault C, Tilkian A, Dement C (1976) The sleep apnoea syndromes. *Ann Rev Med* **27**: 465–84

Haraldsson PO, Carenfelt C, Lysdal M, Tingval C (1995) Does uvulopalatopharyngoplasty inhibit automobile accidents? *Laryngoscope* **105**: 1–5

Hoijer U, Ejnell H, Hedner J, Petruson B, Eng LB (1992) The effect of nasal dilation on snoring and obstructive sleep apnoea. *Arch Otolaryngol Head Neck Surg* **118**(3): 281–4

Hung J, Whitford EG, Parsons RW, Hillman DR (1990) Association of sleep apnea with myocardial infarction in men. *Lancet* **336**: 261–4

Ikeda K, Oshima T, Tanno N et al (1997) Laser-assisted uvulopalatoplasty for habitual snoring without sleep apnea: outcome and complications. *J Otorhinol Rel Special* **59**: 45–9

Ikematsu T (1964) Study of snoring. 4th report: therapy. *J Jap Otorhinolaryngol* **64**: 434–5

Ingrams DR, Spraggs PDR, Pringle MB, Croft CB (1996) $CO_2$ laser palatoplasty: early results. *J Laryngol Otol* **110**: 754–6

Issa FG, Sullivan CE (1984) Upper airway closing pressures in snorers. *J Appl Physiol* **57**: 528–35

Jäger L, Günther E, Gauger J, Reiser M (1998) Fluoroscopic MR of the pharynx in patients with obstructive sleep apnoea. *Am J Neuroradiol* **19**: 1205–14

Jones TM (2005) Unpublished data. MD thesis, University of Liverpool

Jones TM, Ah-See KW (2005) *Surgical and Non-Surgical Interventions for Non-Apnoeic Snoring Patients*. Issue 2. The Cochrane Library. John Wiley and Sons, Chichester

Jones TM, Earis J, Calverley PMA, De S, Swift AC (2005a) Snoring surgery: a retrospective review. *Laryngoscope* (in press)

Jones TM, Swift AC, Calverley PMA, Ho MS, Earis J (2005b) Acoustic analysis of snoring before and after palatal surgery. *Eur Respir J* **25**(6): 1044–9

Kales A, Cadieux RJ, Bixler EO (1985) Severe obstructive sleep apnoea: II. *J Chronic Dis* **38**: 427–34

Kamami Y–V (1990) Laser $CO_2$ for snoring: preliminary results. *Acta Otorhinolaryngol Belg* **44**: 451–6

Katsantonis GP, Schweitzer PK, Branham GH, Chambers G, Walsh JK (1988) Management of obstructive sleep apnea: comparison of various treatment modalities. *Laryngoscope* **98**: 304–9

Koay CB, Freeland AP, Stradling JR (1995) Short- and long-term outcomes of uvulopalatopharyngoplasty for snoring. *Clin Otolaryngol* **20**: 45–8

Koskenvuo M, Kaprio J, Partinen M, Lainginvainio H, Sarna S, Heikkila K (1985) Snoring as a risk factor for hypertension and angina. *Lancet* **i**: 893–6

Koskenvuo M, Kaprio J, Telakivi T, Partinen M, Heikkila K, Sarna S (1987) Snoring as a risk factor for ischemic heart disease and stroke in men. *Br Med J* **294**: 16–18

Krespi YP, Keidar A, Khosh M, Pearlman SJ, Zammit GP (1994) The efficacy of laser-assisted uvulopalatoplasty in the management of obstructive sleep apnea and upper airway resistance syndrome. *Op Tech Otolaryngol Head Neck Surg* **2**: 235–43

Krespi YP, Pearlman SJ (1995) Laser assisted uvulopalatoplasty for the treatment of snoring. *Curr Opin Otolaryngol Head Neck Surg* **3**: 195–200

Lugaresi E, Coccagna G, Cirignotta F (1978) Snoring and its clinical implications. In: Guilleminault C, Dement WC, eds. *Sleep Apnoea Syndrome*. Alan R Liss, New York: 13–21

Mair EA, Day RH (1996) Cautery-assisted palatal stiffening operation. *Otolaryngol Head Neck Surg* **115**: 50

Maniglia AJ (1993) Sleep apnoea and snoring: an overview. *Ear Nose Throat J* **72**: 16–9

Marais J (1998) The value of sedation nasendoscopy: a comparison between snoring and non-snoring patients. *Clin Otolaryngol* **23**: 74–6

McCombe AW, Kwok V, Hawke WM (1995) An acoustic screening test for obstructive sleep apnoea. *Clin Otolaryngol* **20**: 348–51

McGown AD, Makker HK, Battagel JM, L`Estrange PR, Grant HR, Spiro SG (2001) Long-term use of mandibular advancement splints for snoring and obstructive sleep apnoea: a questionnaire suvey. *Eur Resp J* **17**(3): 462–6

Morar P, Nandapalan V, Lesser THJ, Swift AC (1995) Mucosal strip uvulectomy by the $CO_2$ laser as a method of treating simple snoring. *Clin Otolaryngol* **20**: 487

Osborne JE, Osman EZ, Hill PD, Lee BV, Sparkes C (1999) A new acoustic method of differentiating palatal from non-palatal snoring. *Clin Otolaryngol* **24**: 130–3

Partinen M, Palomaki H (1985) Snoring and cerebral infarction. *Lancet* **ii**: 1325–6

Perez-Padilla JR, Slawinski E, Difrancesco LM, Feige RR, Remmers JE, Whitelaw WA (1993) Characteristics of the snoring noise in patients with and without occlusive sleep apnoea. *Am Rev Respir Dis* **147**: 635–44

Prichard AJN, Smithson J, White JES et al (1995) Objective measurement of the results of uvulopalatopharyngoplasty. *Clin Otolaryngol* **20**: 495–8

Pringle MD, Croft CB (1991) A comparison of sleep nasendoscopy and the Müller manoeuvre. *Clin Otolaryngol* **16**: 559–62

Quinn SJ, Daly N, Ellis PDM (1995) Observation of the mechanism of snoring using sleep nasendoscopy. *Clin Otolaryngol* **20**: 360–4

Quinn SJ, Huang L, Ellis PDM, Ffowcs Williams JE (1996) The differentiation of snoring mechanisms using sound analysis. *Clin Otolaryngol* **21**: 119–23

Ryan CF, Lowe AA, Li D, Fleetham JA (1991) Three-dimensional upper airway computed tomography in obstructive sleep apnoea. *Am Rev Respir Dis* **144**: 428–32

Schmidt-Nowara W, Lowe A, Wiegand L, Cartwright R, Perex-Guerra F, Menn S (1995) Oral appliances for the treatment of snoring and sleep apnoea: a review. *Sleep* **118**(6): 501–10

Sharp JF, Jalaludin M, Murray JAM, Maran AGD (1990) The uvulopalatopharyngoplasty operation: the Edinburgh experience. *J R Soc Med* **83**: 569–70

Shepard JW, Thawley SE (1989) Evaluation of the upper airway by computerised tomography inpatients undergoing uvulopalatopharyngoplasty for obstructive sleep apnoea. *Am Rev Respir Dis* **140**: 711–16

Sher AE, Thorpy MJ, Shprintzen RJ, Spielman AJ, Burack B, Mcgregor PA (1985) Predictive value of Müller manoeuvre in selection of patients for uvulopalatopharyngoplasty. *Laryngoscope* **95**: 1483–7

Sher AE, Shprintzen RJ, Thorpy MJ (1986) Endoscopic observation of obstructive sleep apnoea in children with anomalous upper airways: predictive and therapeutic value. *Int J Paediatr Otorhinolaryngol* **11**(2): 135–46

Smithson AJ, White JES, Griffiths CJ et al (1995) Comparison of methods for assessing snoring. *Clin Otolaryngol* **20**: 443–7

Stradling JR, Crosby JH (1991) Predictors and prevalence of obstructive sleep apnoea and snoring in 1001 middle-aged men. *Thorax* **46**(2): 85–90

Stradling JR, Negus TW, Smith D, Langford B (1998) Mandibular advancement devices for the control of snoring. *Eur Respir J* **11**: 447–50

Takeda K (1998) Sleep nasendoscopy and selection of surgical treatments for simple snoring and sleep apnea syndrome. *J Med Soc Toho Univ* **45**(2): 250–9

Tilkian A, Guilleminault C, Shroeder J et al (1977) Sleep-induced apnea syndrome. *Am J Med* **63**: 348–58

Walker RP, Gatti WM, Poirier N, Davis JS (1996) Objective assessment of snoring before and after laser-assisted uvulopalatoplasty. *Laryngoscope* **106**: 1372–7

Wareing M, Mitchell D (1996) Laser-assisted uvulopalatoplasty: an assessment of a technique. *J Laryngol Otol* **110**: 232–6

Weingarten CZ, Raviv G (1995) Evaluation of criteria for uvulopalatoplasty (UPP). Patient selection using acoustic analysis of oronasal respiration (SNAP testing). *J Otolaryngol* **24**(6): 352–7

Weitzman ED, Pollack CP, Borowiecki B et al (1978) The hypersomnia-sleep apnea syndrome: site and mechanism of upper airway obstruction. In: Guilleminault C, Dement WC, eds. *Sleep Apnea Syndromes*. Alan R Liss, New York:

Wenzel M, Schonhofer B, Siemon K, Kohler D (1997) Nasal strips without effect on obstructive sleep apnoea and snoring. *Pneumologic* **51**(12): 1108–10

Wilde AD, Swift AC (1995) A day-case procedure for treating simple snoring. *Clin Otolaryngol* **20**: 486

Woodhead CJ, Davies JE, Allen MB (1991) Obstructive sleep apnea in adults presenting with snoring. *Clin Otolaryngol* **16**: 401–5

Wright J, Dye R (1995) *Systematic Review on Obstructive Sleep Apnoea: its Effect on Health and Benefit of Treatment*. A report by the Yorkshire Collaborating Centre for Health Services Research. Nuffield Institute for Health, Leeds

Yardley MPJ, Clarke RW, Clegg RT (1997) Diathermy palatoplasty: how we do it. *J Otolaryngol* **26**: 284–5

# Chapter 13

# Nasal manifestations of granulomatous disease

*RGM Hughes, A Drake-Lee*

Granulomatous disease frequently affects the head and neck region, particularly the nose and sinuses. This chapter describes the most common infectious and non-infectious conditions and their clinical features.

Infectious granulomatous diseases resulting from tuberculosis (TB) and leprosy have decreased in frequency in the UK in the 20th century, but have returned slightly in the past 10 years (Butt, 1997). Areas with high immigrant populations will encounter these more often. Non-infectious granulomatous diseases, such as Wegener's granulomatosis (WG) and sarcoidosis, have been increasingly recognized. Many granulomatous diseases affect the nose, and this chapter reviews the manifestations of these diseases; *Table 13.1* shows a simple classification. WG and sarcoidosis are the most common granulomatous diseases that affect the nose in the UK; however, worldwide, the infective causes are more common.

### Table 13.1: Classification of nasal granulomata

| **Non-specific** | |
| --- | --- |
| **Non-infectious** | Wegener's granulomatosis |
| | Sarcoidosis |
| | Pyogenic granuloma |
| | Scleroma |
| **Infectious** | Tuberculosis |
| | Leprosy |
| | Syphilis |
| **Maligancy** | Lethal midline granuloma |

# Symptoms and signs

Diagnosis may be difficult because the symptoms and signs are similar and non-specific. The subtle differences can be distinguished with time. Most patients present with nasal obstruction with or without a sero-sanguineous discharge. Frank bleeding may occur if the disease is particularly active. As the respiratory mucosa is destroyed, crusting becomes more of a problem, and this is frequently fetid.

When the diseases go into remission, crusting, scarring and adhesions develop. Skin lesions and destruction are more common in sarcoidosis, TB and leprosy. If the nasal mucosa is destroyed on both sides of the septum, a perforation occurs because the cartilage derives its nutrition from the overlying mucosa. When the destruction is extensive, the septum collapses. Internally granulomata can be seen; they are haemorrhagic in WG and are pale and yellow in sarcoid. The nose is an ideal site for gaining samples for histology and culture. Each disease will be considered in more detail.

# Imaging

Radiographic imaging by computerized tomography (CT) and magnetic resonance imaging (MRI) may show the extent of the disease in the sinuses, but often the changes are non-specific as a result of inflammation. Bone erosion, intracranial and orbital extension are well demonstrated by CT, and this is the first investigation. Extensive bone erosion is more common with a T-cell lymphoma (lethal midline granuloma). MRI in particular shows coincidental changes in otherwise normal sinuses, and so caution is required interpreting these. Fluid or secretions may be differentiated from soft tissue swelling.

# Histology

Nasal biopsies are taken with the aid of a rigid endoscope from the septum, turbinates or any likely area including the post-nasal space. These may be done under local anaesthesia, but if the sinuses are explored a general anaesthetic is preferable. The biopsy size is important, and Del Buono and Flint (1991) have stated that biopsies >5 mm are more helpful in gaining a diagnosis. Multiple biopsies have been advocated, but the authors have never had a positive biopsy without macroscopic evidence of disease. The histological features may be non-specific. Acute and chronic inflammatory changes, namely macrophages, multinucleated giant cells and lymphocytic infiltration, are seen in most conditions.

Vasculitis, mucosal ulceration and necrosis are not found in all cases of WG, and the biopsies need to be interpreted in the light of the clinical picture and other investigations. Sarcoid has less lymphocytic infiltration, and vasculitis should be absent. Features such as Schramm bodies are calcified debris and are more common in sarcoidosis. Previously, a Kveim test could be examined for comparison. Caseation is not always found in TB and is not present in sarcoidosis. Negative staining for *Mycobacterium tuberculosis* does not rule out this. Biopsies need to be deep and may require repeating. The diagnosis of leprosy is made by deep biopsies demonstrating the presence of acid-fast but not alcohol-fast bacilli. A proportion of any biopsy should be sent for culture, but the form must indicate the type of organisms suspected.

## Non-infectious causes of granulomatous disease of the nose

### Wegener's granulomatosis

WG was first described in 1931 by Klinger, and later in a more detailed account by Wegener (1936, 1939). The aetiology is still unknown, but an immunological hypersensitivity reaction is seen as the most likely cause. Until the advent of immunosuppressive therapy, WG was frequently a fatal condition, with mortality rates >90% (Fauci et al, 1983). In its generalized form, the upper and lower airways and renal systems are affected. However, the eyes, skin and nervous system may also be affected (Murty, 1990). More limited forms may affect any of the above systems.

Nasal involvement may be present in any form of the disease, and gives a good clinical guide to the present disease state. Crusting, epistaxis and/or nasal swelling cause obstruction (*Figures 13.1 and 13.2*).

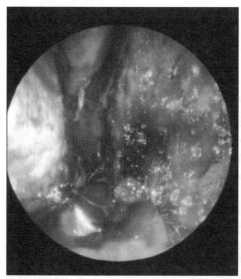

Figure 13.1: Crusting associated with Wegener's granulomatosis.

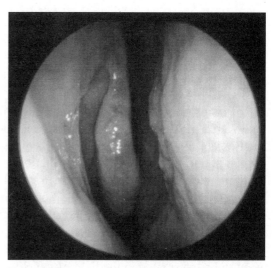

Figure 13.2: Normal nose for comparison with Figure 13.1.

Ulceration and septal perforation are common intranasal findings. Externally, there can be cosmetic changes as a result of the degree of internal destruction. Septal collapse is shown in *Figure 13.3*.

Cutaneous involvement in WG is uncommon, but is more common with sarcoidosis. The presence of gross destruction of the skin means that an alternative diagnosis such as lymphoma should be considered (see later).

Cytoplasmic pattern anti-neutrophil cytoplasmic antibody (c-ANCA) is increasingly playing an important role in the diagnosis and monitoring of the disease process. Rao et al (1995) have shown that the sensitivity and specificity are high in acute disease (91% and 99%, respectively), but this falls in inactive disease (63% and 99.5%, respectively).

### Sarcoidosis

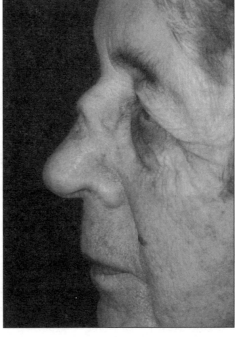

Figure 13.3: Septal collapse (saddling) as a result of Wegener's granulomatosis.

Sarcoidosis is a disease characterized by non-caseating granuloma, with an unknown aetiology. Sarcoidosis is a systemic condition and can affect any tissue; but it has a predilection for lymph nodes, lung and skin. The condition was reviewed recently but excluded essentially the ear, nose and throat manifestations of the disease (Hunninghake et al, 1999). Jonathon Hutchinson described the skin manifestations first in 1877, and Caesar Boeck first described sarcoidosis in 1899, noting both nasal and skin lesions. When nasal sarcoid is present, there is a worse prognosis with the worry that the lesions will spread into the cranial cavity (Hunninghake et al, 1999). The overall mortality of the condition is 5%, and this is associated with the cardiac, renal and intra-cranial spread.

Nasal disease usually manifests its presence by nasal obstruction, epistaxis and rhinorrhoea or postnasal drip. The nasal mucosal appearance is classically 'cobble-stoned' (*Figure 13.4*). The granulomata are distinguished from those in WG, being less haemorrhagic.

Other signs include nasal polyps, crusting, perforation, adhesions, saddling and mucosal oedema.

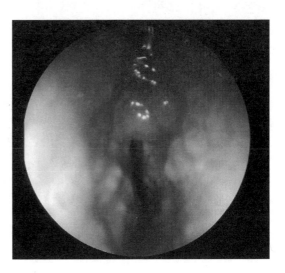

Figure 13.4: Cobble-stone appearance of the nasal mucosa affected by sarcoidosis.

Cutaneous involvement is more common in sarcoidosis, being either the direct involvement of the skin with granulomatous disease or as 'lupus pernio', where deeper granulomas in the dermis produce red or violet skin lesions (*Figure 13.5a,b*).

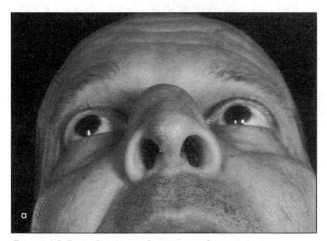
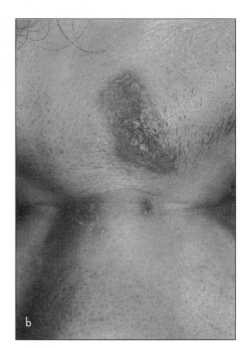

Figure 13.5a,b: Skin manifestations of sarcoidosis.

## Pyogenic granuloma

Pyogenic granuloma (lobular capillary haemangioma) often present as an alarming, rapidly enlarging, unilateral nasal mass causing epistaxis and nasal blockage. This problem is uncommon, but occurs through the age ranges and is seen in children. A history of trauma is not always given, but is almost always the cause, and treatment is surgical excision. Recurrence is uncommon (el-Sayed and al-Serhani, 1997).

## Scleroma

Scleroma is a chronic granulomatous condition, which is slowly progessive. Typically, the disease is present initally in the nose but then extends into the nasopharynx, oropharynx and larynx. This condition is rare in the UK. It is more common in the subtropics and the Middle East. The causative organism is *Klesbiella rhinoscleroma*. Three clinical stages have been described:

* catarrhal rhinitis
* inflammatory granulomatous
* cicatricial deformation.

The first stage gives symptoms similar to a cold; the second nasal blockage, ulceration and foul discharge; the third produces disfigurement.

# Infectious causes of granulomatous diseases of the nose

## Tuberculosis

Classically there are two forms of TB of the nose:

⌘ lupus vulgaris
⌘ granulomatous TB.

It is a rare condition, with only 35 cases being reported in the English language medical literature in the last 95 years (Butt, 1997), although clearly the disease is more common in the non-English speaking world. Lupus vulgaris is a destructive skin lesion, which may involve the nasal vestibule; granulomatous TB involves the anterior nasal septum rather than the skin, producing nasal obstruction and foul-smelling discharge. The bony septum is not involved, and cosmetically unappealing scarring may occur after the initial ulceration. Atrophic rhinitis is a frequent sequel. There is confusion regarding whether nasal TB is strongly associated with pulmonary TB.

## Leprosy

Leprosy produces a wide range of clinical features dependent upon the host immunological reaction to the intracellular *Mycobacterium leprae*. The lepromatous form produces large quantities of mycobacterium, as opposed to the tuberculoid leprosy where the numbers of organisms may be small. Nasal discharge is a potent method by which leprosy is spread. Skin involvement is frequent in leprosy, and the nose is often the first site involved. Clinical features are granulomatous nodules, perforation and ulceration on the septum and turbinates. These tend to heal, producing atrophic rhinitis. There has been one documented case presenting to an ear, nose and throat department in Birmingham in the past 10 years, and as expected it occurred in an immigrant.

## Syphilis

Syphilis has decreased in frequency with increasing antibiotic usage, but should always be considered in a case of granulomatous nasal disease. Transmission is either congenital or acquired. Recently there has been an increase in the reported prevalence, particularly epidemics occurring in Russia, and within the male homosexual community (Borisenko et al, 1999). In congenital syphilis, the nose is always involved and causes discharge that may be present at birth. The erythematous patches of secondary syphilis tend to develop within the next 3–6 months. This chronic discharge is thick, yellow and blood stained. Tertiary syphilis causes nasal deformity, collapse of the bridge of the nose, perforation of the hard palate and septum and ulceration of the nasal skin.

Acquired syphilis first gives a primary chancre of the nose, usually of the vestibule or anterior part of the septum. Cervical lymphadenopathy is not uncommon. Secondary syphilis then develops and is similar to the ulceration seen in the other orifices such as the mouth. Tertiary syphilis develops to give the characteristic saddle deformity (as a result of nasal bone destruction, not septal perforation), and granulomatous lesions in the nose with ulceration. A posterior septal perforation is associated with syphilis, whereas an anterior perforation is not caused by syphilis. The destruction by tertiary syphilis may be expansive and cause bone necrosis.

TB, leprosy and syphilis are the commonest infectious causes of granulomatous disease, but there are other rare causes, including Yaws, actinomycosis, nocardiosis and some fungal infections, especially aspergillosis, leishmaniasis and Churg–Strauss disease (allergic granulomatosis). All are rare, but should be considered in the differential diagnosis.

### Lethal midline granuloma (Stewart's granuloma)

Lethal midline granuloma is a misnomer; the condition is a nasal T-cell lymphoma (*Figure 13.6*).

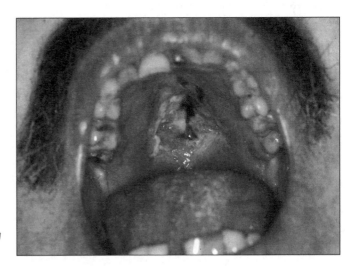

*Figure 13.6: Palatal destruction as a result of a lymphoma.*

This is an extremely destructive lesion of the mid-face and requires a biopsy for diagnosis; these may require repeating.

The treatment is radiotherapy, but cure is not guaranteed.

Previously 'midline destructive lesions' of the sinonasal tract had a variety of terms, including midfacial destructive lesion, Stewart's granuloma and midline malignant reticulosis, but probably represent the lymphoma described previously (Harrison, 1987). However, recent studies have again suggested that 'idiopathic midline destructive disease' is still a valid description/diagnosis for a few patients where other diagnoses have been excluded (Barker and Hosni, 1998).

# Conclusion

The nose is part of the respiratory tract and may be involved in any systemic disease that affects any part of it. WG has a predilection for presenting with nasal symptoms. While in the UK, the causes are usually WG or sarcoidosis; worldwide, infection remains the commonest cause. The role of the ear, nose and throat surgeon is to help make the diagnosis and monitor the progress of the condition, and therapy is best left to those who specialize in medical treatment.

# References

Barker TH, Hosni AA (1998) Idiopathic midline destructive disease — does it exist? *J Laryn Otol* **112**(3): 307–9

Borisenko KK, Tichonova LI, Renton AM (1999) Syphilis and other sexually transmitted infections in the Russian Federation. *Int J STD AIDS* **10**(10): 665–8

Butt AA (1997) Nasal tuberculosis in the 20th century. *Am J Med Sci* **313**(6): 332–5

Del Buono EA, Flint A (1991) Diagnostic usefulness of nasal biopsy in Wegener's granulomatosis. *Hum Pathol* **22**(2): 107–10

Fauci AS, Hayes BF, Katz P et al (1983) Wegener's granulomatosis. Prospective clinical and therapeutic experience with 85 patients for 21 years. *Ann Intern Med* **98**: 76–85

el-Sayed Y, al-Serhani A (1997) Lobular capillary haemangioma (pyogenic granuloma) of the nose. *J Laryn Otol* **11**(10): 941–5

Klinger H (1931) Grenzformen der Periarteritis Nodosa. *Z Pathol* **42**: 455–80

Harrison DFN (1987) Midline destructive granuloma: fact or fiction? *Laryngoscope* **97**: 1049–53

Hunninghake G, Costabel U, Ando K et al (1999) AST/ERS/WASOG statement on sarcoidosis. *Sarcoidosis Vasc Diffuse Lung Dis* **16**: 149–73

Murty GE (1990) Wegener's granulomatosis: otorhinolaryngological manifestations. *Clin Otol* **15**: 385–93

Rao JK, Weinberger M, Oddone EZ, Allen NB, Landsman P, Feussner JR (1995) The role of antineutrophil cytoplasmic cytoplasmic antibody (c-ANCA) testing in the diagnosis of Wegener granulomatosis. A literature review and meta-analysis. *Ann Int Med* **123**(12): 925–32

Wegener F (1936) Uber generalisierte Septische Grefassenkrankungen. *Verh Dtsch Ges Pathol* **29**: 202–10

Wegener F (1939) Ubeer eine Eigenartige Rhinogene granulomatose mit besonderer Beteiligung des Arteriensystems und der nieren. *Beitr Pathol* **102**: 168–79

# Chapter 14

# The case for a one-stop balance centre

*Jim Cook*

Vertigo, imbalance and dizziness are poorly understood symptoms. This lack of understanding often results in a feeling of therapeutic impotence and frustration. Despair may be felt by the treating physician and hence the patient. This is particularly unfortunate because most patients with imbalance can be helped, often on a single-visit basis.

Vertigo and imbalance can be extremely debilitating symptoms. They frequently result in a tendency to fall and a fear of leaving the home environment. Serious injuries may occur in the elderly, including fractures of the neck of femur and radius and head trauma often resulting in long-term hospital admission, institutionalization and even death.

It is estimated that falls are the main cause of death from injuries in those over 65 years old. Dizziness becomes increasingly common with age, and the incidence is rising as the longevity of populations within developed countries rises (Kroenke and Manglesdorff, 1989; Herdman, 1994). As balance disorders are likely to increase the probability of a fall and subsequent injury, it would seem that the management of dizziness in the elderly should be a healthcare priority (Campbell et al, 1981; Prudem and Evans, 1981; Blake et al, 1988; Tinnetti et al, 1988). Unfortunately, this problem is not as yet generally recognized.

The problem is not confined to the elderly. In younger adults, unemployment and the withdrawal of a driving licence are serious risks. The ability to look after a young child may be impaired and family stability jeopardized.

Patients with dizziness are often misunderstood, as they find it difficult to describe their symptoms. The commonest description is perhaps of light-headedness or a feeling of being under the influence of alcohol. A sensation of violent rotation may also occur. More abstract descriptions are often heard, such as 'a sensation of water running down inside the head', 'cotton wool in the head', 'not quite being there' and 'not being able to catch up with my environment'. This may lead to a misunderstanding on the part of the clinician and a sense of frustration for both the clinician and the patient.

It is therefore not surprising that dizzy patients are on the whole not popular with the medical fraternity. This is particularly unfortunate as dizziness is extremely common. In the USA, 30% of the population have experienced episodes of dizziness by the age of 65 years (Roydhouse, 1974).

# Causes of dizziness

While there are cardiovascular and neurological causes for dizziness, by far the majority of patients have abnormalities of their vestibular apparatus. It is useful to understand why patients feel dizzy. The principal cause is abnormal eye movements that occur as a consequence of head movements. In health, head movements stimulate the vestibular apparatus so that optic fixation may be obtained on a target when the head moves. Abnormalities of these vestibular-ocular reflexes (VORs) result in retinal slippage, which induces a sensation of movement (oscillopsia). Such abnormalities can arise as a result of lesions anywhere in the network connecting the vestibular apparatus through the brainstem to the external ocular muscles. However, the commonest causes lie within the labyrinth.

An individual may feel that their environment has moved when it has not. If these inappropriate eye movements are subtle, a sensation of light-headedness may be experienced, but if they are more severe, a sensation of rotation will be felt. When VORs are abnormal, a patient may substitute other senses to retain their balance. These include the use of proprioception and vision. When standing on an unstable surface or in the dark, the latter two senses become ineffective and the individual has to rely upon their vestibular apparatus. If this does not occur, there is an increased likelihood of falling.

Visual preference is a particular problem and occurs when undue reliance is put upon vision as opposed to proprioception and vestibular function. A frequently experienced example occurs when sitting in a train adjacent to another train. When the second train moves, it is common to sense movement of the train in which the observer is sitting. In health, the lack of vestibular stimulation, because the observer is not moving quickly, overcomes this impression and the illusion is usually only momentary. With a vestibular disorder, this impression may be prolonged because of a preference to substitute visual information for vestibular.

# Diagnostic issues in vertigo

Some specific diagnoses of vertigo are particularly important to identify, as they require specific treatment. Benign paroxysmal positional vertigo occurs as a result of stimulation of the ampulla, usually of the posterior semicircular canal when the head is turned 45° to the affected side, with the individual supine. In this position, the posterior semicircular canal is in a vertical position. Gravitational stimulation of this ampulla, perhaps by calcium particles released from the otoconia within the utricle (cupulolithiasis) or the semicircular canals (canalolithiasis) results in upward movement of the eyes with a rebound, down-beating nystagmus. It is possible to reposition these particles into the utricle by means of manoeuvres such as the Epley manoeuvre.

An unpublished audit of the results achieved by this manoeuvre at the Leicester Balance Centre has revealed symptomatic resolution of positional vertigo in 75% of cases following one manoeuvre and 95% following two manoeuvres. However, some patients subsequently develop imbalance on head movement, although they usually respond to a customized vestibular rehabilitation (VR) programme.

Ménière's disease consists of a triad of symptoms, including vertigo, tinnitus and hearing loss, which is sometimes associated with aural fullness. It may be amenable to treatment with a low-salt and low-caffeine diet and surgical procedures, including grommet insertion, labyrinthectomy, endolymphatic sac surgery and, most recently, perfusion of the cochlea with gentamicin or steroids.

Central causes of vertigo need to be identified, thus a magnetic resonance imaging (MRI) scan should be ordered. Conversely, if a lesion can be shown to be peripheral, an MRI scan can be avoided.

Other specific diagnoses are not so important as treatment will usually take the form of VR. In a second unpublished audit at the Leicester Balance Centre, it was found that 85% of patients received an 80% resolution of their symptoms after VR treatment as assessed by the Dizziness Handicap Inventory (Jacobsen and Newman, 1990).

## Referral patterns

A third internal audit recently took place at Leicester Royal Infirmary to establish how patients with imbalance were investigated and treated. A typical pattern would be for patients to present to their GP. Most patients would not receive a secondary referral. Those that were referred would often present to a neurologist, general physician, care of the elderly specialist or a general ear, nose and throat (ENT) consultant.

On average, the audit found that a dizzy patient would see five physicians before receiving a specific treatment targeted at their condition. Multiple investigations were often organized, including MRI, 24-hour electrocardiographic monitoring and tilt-table testing, which were all usually within normal limits. Should all these investigations be ordered, the typical interval between a patient first presenting to the GP and receiving treatment, usually in the form of VR, could be up to 3 years. In the USA, a solution to this problem was found by setting up single-visit balance centres. Within these centres, a patient would undergo a consultation, receive the appropriate investigations and have their treatment organized and instituted in a single sitting. This is a model that has been adopted at the Leicester Balance Centre, but surprisingly at no other unit within the UK as at present.

## The case for a one-stop balance clinic

It is clear from the above that there are savings to be made in terms of finance and morbidity by running a one-stop balance clinic. However, as has been indicated, imbalance is a common symptom, and there may be a reluctance to offer such a service because of the demands that it may create. Conversely, if falls can be prevented in the elderly, emergency admissions as a result of trauma could potentially be reduced, leading to a huge reduction in financial demands made upon the health service.

The Leicester Balance Centre was opened following visits to Dr Neil Shepard's balance unit at Ann Arbor University in Michigan and Dr Joel Goebel's unit at the University of Washington, St Louis, USA. Clearly, the healthcare systems in the USA and UK are different, and it was not immediately clear how to adopt the business plans that they had used (available from SLE, Croydon, Surrey) for the purposes of the Leicester Balance Centre. Nevertheless, common ground was found. A proposal was made to Leicester Royal Infirmary to run a one-stop unit on a partially self-funding basis. By treating both NHS and private patients, income was generated for the purchase of equipment and for the funding of staff. A case was also made for the reduction in the number of potentially expensive and inappropriate investigations that might otherwise be performed.

Three aspects of setting up the service were identified, namely the requirements for staff, space and equipment. Since VR is the cornerstone of the treatment of most dizzy patients, physiotherapy resources are essential. Before setting up the unit, rehabilitation was available through the hospital physiotherapy unit and usually took the form of Cawthorne Cooksey exercises. However, a delay of up to 1 year in patients being seen was usual.

It is known that customized rehabilitation is significantly more effective than Cawthorne Cooksey exercises, particularly when performed by a physiotherapist with a particular interest in rehabilitation (Shumway-Cook and Horak, 1990; Shepard et al, 1993; Shepard and Telian, 1995). It was therefore decided to recruit a vestibular physiotherapist to be employed directly by the ENT department.

With respect to equipment, computerized electronystagmography and audiometry were already available, but there was no facility for looking at other aspects of imbalance, such as sensory organization (the appropriate use of vestibular, visual and proprioceptive senses) and motor control function. Both of these areas can be investigated by means of computerized dynamic posturography, and an Equitest machine (NeuroCom, Clackamas, Oregon, USA) was purchased (*Figure 14.1*).

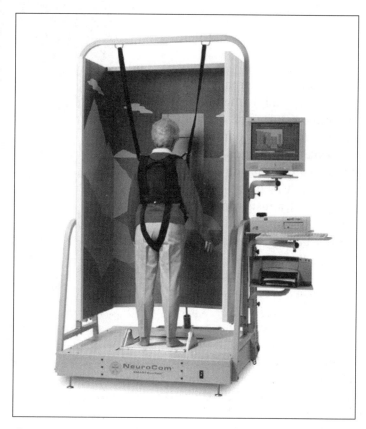

*Figure 14.1: Computerized dynamic posturography being performed on the Equitest (NeuroCom, Clackamas, Oregon, USA). Appropriate use of vestibular, visual and proprioceptive senses can be examined, together with the patient's ability to maintain balance using motor control.*

The time of a consultant ENT surgeon was made available by dividing a pre-existing ENT clinic into three 1-hour sessions, all beginning at 8.30 am, and six patients per session were examined. The appropriate tests were ordered, performed after the consultation and the patient reviewed after the tests. VR, if appropriate, was then planned and the patient kept under review by the vestibular physiotherapist at approximately monthly intervals until symptomatic resolution occurred. Support by telephone to the patient was made available, which helped reduce the number of follow-up visits.

In the first year, the centre saw over 1000 new patients. Perhaps not surprisingly, the centre has proved increasingly popular, and in January 2001 it increased its capacity to involve a further clinician and physiotherapist to cope with the anticipated demand of nearly 2000 new patients a year. Future developments include the acquisition of a computerized infrared oculography system to compliment the current electronystagmography equipment (*Figure 14.2*) and high-speed vestibular acceleration testing.

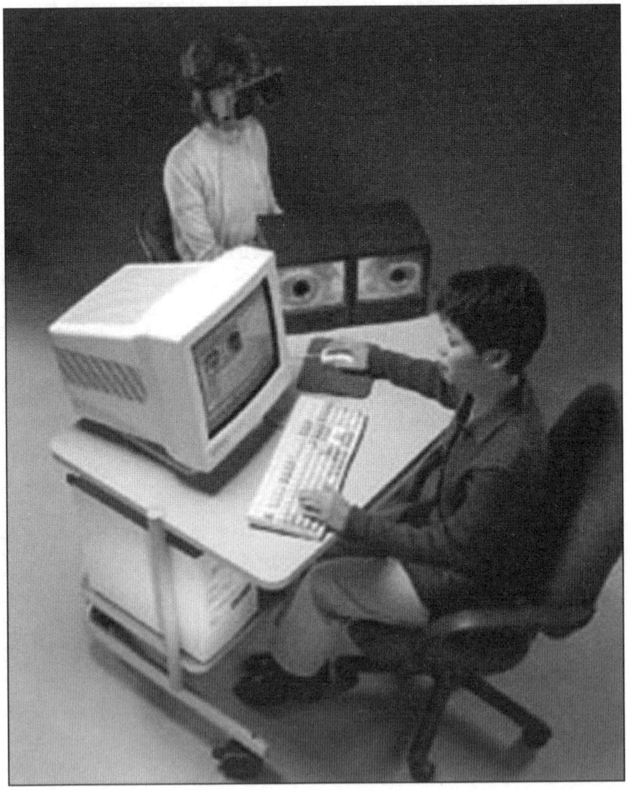

*Figure 14.2: Computerized infrared oculography system used to examine vestibular-ocular reflex function.*

Technicians from the hearing services and medical physics departments have now been multiskilled so that they can perform all the tests available. Technicians are involved in the initial consultation and planning of treatment, which provide staff with a much greater insight into the rationale for performing the investigations. Technicians can then follow the patients through their tests and become involved in their treatment, to the benefit of both technician and patient alike.

It is clear that this approach has required significant changes in working practices. As is usual with change, members of staff expressed misgivings. However, the openness with which the service was set up and the degree of inclusivity and ownership given to all staff have helped to minimize these fears.

Combined clinics with the departments of neurology and dietetics (chiefly for treating patients with Ménière's disease) are also run.

Referrals are now received; not only from Leicestershire, but also from throughout the UK, Europe and beyond.

Visits to the department are welcome by arrangement.

# References

Blake AJ, Morgan K, Bendall MJ et al (1988) Falls by elderly people at home: prevalence and associated factors. *Age Ageing* **17**: 365–72

Campbell AJ, Reinken J, Allan BC, Martinez GS (1981) Falls in old age: a study of frequency and related clinical factors. *Age Ageing* **10**: 264–70

Herdman SJ (1994) *Vestibular Rehabilitation*. FA Davis Co, Philadelphia: ix–x

Jacobsen GP, Newman CW (1990) The development of the dizziness handicap inventory. *Arch Otolaryngol Head Neck Surg* **116**: 424–7

Kroenke K, Manglesdorff AG (1989) Common symptoms in ambulatory care: incidence, evaluation, therapy and outcome. *Am J Med* **86**: 262–6

Prudem G, Evans J (1981) Factors associated with falls in the elderly: a community study. *Age Ageing* **10**: 141–6

Roydhouse N (1974) Vertigo and its treatment. *Drugs* **7**: 297–309

Shepard NT, Telian SA (1995) Programmatic vestibular rehabilitation. *Otolaryngol Head Neck Surg* **112**: 173–82

Shepard NT, Telian SA, Smith-Wheelock M, Raj A (1993) Vestibular and balance rehabilitation therapy. *Ann Otol Rhinol Laryngol* **102**: 198–205

Shumway-Cook A, Horak FB (1990). Rehabilitation strategies for patients with vestibular deficits. *Neurol Clin* **8**: 441–57

Tinnetti ME, Speechlay M, Ginter SF (1988) Risk factors for falls among elderly persons living in the community. *N Engl J Med* **319**: 1701–7

# Chapter 15

# Balance disorders in adults: an overview

*R Palaniappan*

Dizziness is a common and potentially disabling complaint. A multitude of medical and otological conditions may manifest as disequilibrium. Symptomatic improvement in peripheral vestibular lesion is the result of central compensation and not restoration of normal labyrinthine function.

Dizziness is a non-specific symptom, which does not instantly point to any specific organ systems. Disequilibrium may result from disturbance in a number of structures, including the visual, proprioceptive, vestibular, cardiovascular and central nervous system. Each year, 5 out of every 1000 patients consult their GP for vertigo, and a further 10 in 1000 are seen for dizziness or giddiness (Royal College of General Practitioners and Office of Population Census and Surveys, 1986). The term dizziness is commonly used interchangeably to describe four categories of balance dysfunction: vertigo, disequilibrium or unsteadiness, near-syncope and non-specific light-headedness.

## What is vertigo?

Vertigo is defined as an illusion or hallucination of movement, and is typically thought to arise from an abnormality involving the peripheral or central vestibular pathways (*Figure 15.1*).

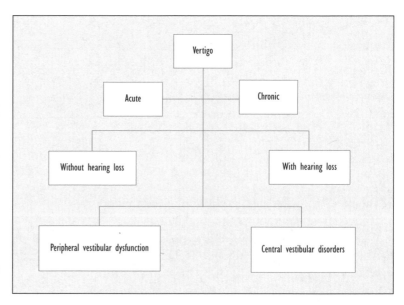

*Figure 15.1: Classification of vertigo.*

A clear-cut distinction should therefore be made between vertigo and non-specific light-headedness, dizziness or faintness, which may be caused by a plethora of general medical conditions. A carefully obtained thorough history, combined with targeted physical examination, would pave the way for successful diagnosis in the majority of instances.

Dizziness is a common but often untreated symptom, which is associated with extensive handicap and psychological morbidity (Yardley et al, 1998). It is important to realize that not all dizziness is vertigo, even though patients may describe vertigo as dizziness. It is therefore useful to ask the patient to describe the exact sensation and any other associated symptoms, such as nausea, vomiting or headache.

## Classification of vertigo

The history usually provides the vital information necessary to distinguish peripheral from central causes of vertigo (Baloh, 1998) (*Table 15.1*).

**Table 15.1: Historical features that would help distinguish peripheral from central vertigo**

| Features | Peripheral | Central |
| --- | --- | --- |
| Imbalance | Mild–moderate | Severe |
| Nausea and vomiting | Severe | Variable (may be minimal) |
| Auditory symptoms | Common | Rare |
| Neurological symptoms | Rare | Common |
| Compensation | Rapid | Slow |

Adapted from Baloh and Honrubia (1990)

The history should include:

⌘ The mode of onset and description of the first episode
⌘ Frequency and duration of individual attack
⌘ Whether it is spontaneous or provoked by certain factors, such as head movement
⌘ Associated auditory symptoms, such as hearing loss or tinnitus
⌘ Head trauma
⌘ Concomitant ear disease or previous aural surgery.

When the symptoms are global and the patient describes the sensation as 'wooziness', being 'about to blackout' or 'disoriented', a presyncopal cause secondary to insufficient blood flow to the central nervous system is assumed.

More than one factor may contribute to balance disorder in the elderly, such as visual and proprioceptive disturbance. In some patients, an accurate diagnosis may emerge only after a period of review.

## Peripheral *vs* central vestibular dysfunction

Vertigo may present as:

⌘ A spontaneous attack with prolonged recovery lasting days
⌘ Recurrent attacks lasting minutes to hours
⌘ Brief attacks induced by position change, usually lasting less than a minute.

A peripheral or a central disorder may cause each of these syndromes. Gait unsteadiness and fear of falling are more common manifestations of neurological disorders. Patients with a history of falls require thorough evaluation of risk factors, such as drug intake, neurological condition, cognitive function, environmental factors and general medical conditions (*Figure 15.2*).

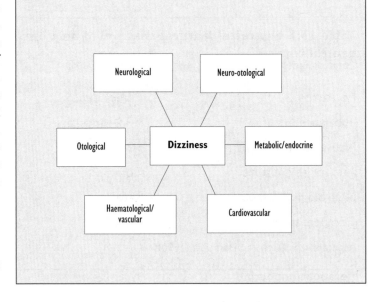

*Figure 15.2: Causes of dizziness in adults.*

Disorders affecting the peripheral vestibular system often cause associated hearing impairment. However, conditions such as benign paroxysmal positional vertigo (BPPV), vestibular neuronitis and familial vestibulopathy selectively affect the peripheral vestibular system without causing hearing loss.

Bath et al (2000) report peripheral vestibulopathy as the cause of dizziness in 64.7% of adults, with central, psychiatric and unknown causes respectively accounting for 8.1%, 9% and 13.3% of cases (*Table 15.2*).

# Table 15.2: Aetiology of dizziness in adults

| Systems | Conditions |
| --- | --- |
| **Otological** | Benign paroxysmal positional vertigo |
| | Labyrinthitis |
| | Ménière's disease |
| | Ototoxic drugs |
| | Vestibular neuronitis |
| | Otosyphillis |
| | Cholesteatoma |
| | Perilymph fistula |
| **Neuro-otological** | Cerebello-pontine angle tumours |
| | Vestibular schwannoma |
| | Meningioma |
| | Metastatic tumours |
| | Arachnoid cysts |
| **Neurological** | Multiple sclerosis |
| | Parkinson's disease |
| | Cerebellar or brainstem infarction |
| | Syncope |
| **Cardiovascular** | Aortic stenosis |
| | Carotid sinus hypersensitivity |
| | Cardiac dysrhythmias |
| **Haematological** | Anaemia |
| | Hyperviscosity syndrome |
| | Leukaemias |
| | Sickle cell disease |
| **Vascular** | Autoimmune vasculitis |
| | Carotid artery stenosis |
| | Vertebrobasilar ischaemia |
| | Subclavian steal syndrome |
| **Metabolic/endocrine** | Hyper-/hypoglycaemia |
| | Hyperventilation |
| | Thyroid disease |
| **Others** | Psychological disorders |
| | Cervical vertigo |
| | Visual vertigo |
| | Head injury |
| | Drug induced, other than ototoxic medications |
| | Multisensory dizziness syndrome |
| | Chronic fatigue syndrome |

Duration of the individual attack will usually give an idea about the possible underlying pathology.

Sudden rotatory vertigo of less than a minute is commonly caused by BPPV, whereas vertigo of several hours is a manifestation of Ménière's disease or migraine.

In between attacks, there may be periods of long remission. A single, acute episode of vertigo with gradual improvement in symptoms is most commonly the result of an acute peripheral vestibular event, such as viral or ischaemic labyrinthitis. Patients with poorly compensated peripheral vestibular disorder may complain of constant disequilibrium, which in the absence of an acute attack should prompt a search for central vestibular pathology.

## Vertigo associated with hearing loss

Vertigo associated with hearing loss may be a manifestation of Ménière's disease, temporal bone fracture, otitic barotrauma, perilymph fistula, vestibular schwannoma, labyrinthitis, otosyphilis, ototoxic drugs and autoimmune inner-ear disease.

## Benign paroxysmal positional vertigo

BPPV is one of the most common causes (25%) of dizziness (Epley, 1996) and is thought to arise from the presence of abnormal dense particles, most likely otoconial debris, in the long arm of the posterior semicircular canal. BPPV is characterized by severe paroxysms of rotational vertigo provoked by positional changes of the head. Dix and Hallpike's positional test, which provokes dizziness and a typical geotropic nystagmus, is diagnostic of BPPV (Epley, 1995). It is eminently treatable by a canalith repositioning procedure.

## Vestibular neuronitis

Vestibular neuronitis is reportedly the third most common cause of peripheral vestibular vertigo following BPPV and Ménière's disease (Strupp and Brandt, 1999). Sudden onset of severe vertigo with nausea, vomiting and absence of auditory symptoms typify vestibular neuronitis.

# Cervical vertigo

Lack of definite diagnostic tests makes cervical vertigo a controversial clinical entity. Vertigo associated with neck movements could result from disorders of vestibular, visual, vascular, neurovascular or cervico-proprioceptive mechanisms. The proponents of this condition claim that dizziness of cervical origin could result from cervical tone imbalance, secondary to defective neck proprioceptors. However, such a tone imbalance has not been demonstrated in whiplash injuries or cervical pain syndromes. Nevertheless, if true cervical vertigo exists, the treatment is similar to that of the underlying neck condition (Brandt and Bronstein, 2001).

# Bilateral vestibular failure

Bilateral vestibular failure (BVF) may present with recurrent episodes of vertigo associated with unsteadiness in the dark and ossilopsia on head movement. Ototoxic drugs, such as gentamycin, commonly cause BVF, which is often associated with some degree of high-frequency sensorineural hearing loss. Approximately 20% of patients with BVF have no identifiable cause (Rinne et al, 1998). Management of patients with bilateral vestibular loss is difficult; the emphasis is on maximizing and optimizing visual and proprioceptive inputs. Patients should be counselled regarding safety considerations, such as night-lights at home or assistive devices, and should be warned of the risk of drowning while diving. Familial vestibulopathy without hearing loss may be inherited as an autosomal dominant condition (Baloh et al, 1994).

# Compensation

Compensation is a central process, therefore peripheral lesions tend to compensate more readily than brainstem or cerebellar causes. About 80% of patients respond favourably to vestibular rehabilitation exercises (Luxon, 1998).

# Inadequate/poor compensation

Vestibular sedatives are useful adjuncts in the management of acute vertigo, but their long-term use may delay compensation. Other causes of poorly compensated vestibular dysfunction include inappropriate exercise strategy, poor vision and psychological factors (*Table 15.3*).

## Table 15.3: Aetiology of poor compensation in peripheral vestibular dysfunction

| | |
|---|---|
| **Drug-related factors** | Prolonged use of vestibular sedatives, tranquillisers and other psychotropic drugs |
| | Strong hypotensives |
| | Anticonvulsant use may need to be reviewed and balanced |
| **Psychological factors** | Avoidance behaviour |
| | Anxiety, depression and panic attacks |
| **Visual problems** | New glasses: bifocals, change of prescription |
| | Development of cataract |
| | Retinopathy: diabetes mellitus, hypertension |
| | Macular degeneration |
| **Musculoskeletal disorders** | Stiff or painful neck or back |
| | Arthritis of major weight-bearing joints |
| **Neurological disorders** | Neuropathy: diabetes mellitus, alcohol |
| | Recent posterior circulation infarction |
| **Cardiovascular causes** | Poorly controlled or untreated hypertension |
| | Arrhythmias |
| | Valvular heart disease |
| | Inadequate cardiac output as a result of other medical |
| **Haematological problems** | Anaemia |
| | Polycythaemia rubra vera |
| **Vestibular factors** | Progressive peripheral vestibular dysfunction: Ménière's disease |
| | Bilateral vestibular failure |
| | Concomitant untreated benign paroxysmal positional vertigo |
| | New central vestibular disorder: multiple sclerosis, cerebellar atrophy |
| **Exercise-related factors** | Inappropriate exercise regimens |
| | Poor motivation and compliance |

# Central vertigo

Common central causes of recurrent, spontaneous vertigo are migraine and vertebrobasilar transient ischaemia. A family history is helpful in supporting a diagnosis of vestibular migraine. Common central causes of a single attack of vertigo lasting more than 24 hours include posterior circulation infarction, cerebellar or brainstem haemorrhage and multiple sclerosis (Solomon, 2000). Brainstem and cerebellar lesions can cause a persistent positional vertigo with down beat, up beat or torsional nystagmus.

Imbalance in the absence of typical vertigo may be seen in patients with bilateral vestibular loss, significant peripheral neuropathy (diabetes) or spinal cord dorsal column lesions (compressive, vitamin $B_{12}$ deficiency, syphilis). Other causes include cerebellar atrophy, white matter disease, normal pressure hydrocephalus and extrapyramidal disorders (Parkinson's disease, progressive supranuclear palsy). Patients with recurrent or persistent vertigo of more than 6 weeks' duration should be investigated neuro-otologically (Luxon, 1997).

## Investigation of dizziness

Investigation of the dizzy patient may include some or all of the following tests based on history and clinical findings (*Table 15.4*).

### Table 15.4: Investigations for dizziness

| | |
|---|---|
| **Audio-vestibular** | Pure tone audiogram |
| | Stapedial reflexes |
| | Auditory brainstem responses |
| | Electronystagmography |
| | Posturography (Equitest, Neurocom International, Clackamas, Oregon, USA) |
| | Caloric test |
| **Haematological/ biochemical** | Full blood count |
| | Urea and electrolytes |
| | Fasting blood sugar |
| | Serum lipids |
| | Thyroid function tests |
| | Serology for syphilis |
| | Autoimmune profile |
| **Radiological** | Magnetic resonance imaging |
| | X-ray cervical spine |
| | Magnetic resonance angiography |
| | Transcranial Doppler ultrasound |

A magnetic resonance imaging brain scan may be required to rule out cerebello-pontine angle tumours, such as vestibular schwannoma. Transcranial Doppler ultrasound is becoming increasingly popular in the evaluation of vascular dizziness.

## Conclusion

Dizziness is a vague symptom, which may be a manifestation of wide-ranging pathological processes. Chronic episodic vertigo resulting from inadequately compensated peripheral vestibular disorder is an important cause of morbidity and time taken out of work. Rehabilitation of patients with peripheral vestibular dysfunction is aimed at improving central compensation by means of physiotherapeutic measures with or without medical and or psychotherapeutic intervention.

## References

Baloh RW, Honrubia V (1990) *Clinical Neurophysiology of the Vestibular System.* 2nd edn. FA Davies, Philadelphia

Baloh RW, Jacobson K, Fife T (1994) Familial vestibulopathy: a new dominantly inherited syndrome. *Neurology* **44**: 20–5

Baloh RW (1998) Differentiating between peripheral and central causes of vertigo. *Otolaryngol Head Neck Surg* **119**: 55–9

Bath AP, Walsh RM, Ranalli P et al (2000) Experience from a multidisciplinary 'dizzy' clinic. *Am J Otol* **21**: 92–7

Brandt T, Bronstein AM (2001) Cervical vertigo. *J Neuro Neurosurg Psychiatry* **71**: 8–12

Epley JM (1995) Positional vertigo related to semicircular canalithiasis. *Otolaryngol Head Neck Surg* **112**(1): 155–61

Epley JM (1996) Particle repositioning for benign paroxysmal positional vertigo. *Otolaryngol Clin North Am* **29**(2): 323–31

Luxon LM (1997) The medical management of vertigo. *J Otol Laryngol* **111**: 1114–21

Luxon LM (1998) Assessment and management of vertigo. *Prescribers' J* **38**(2): 87–97

Rinne T, Bronstein AM, Rudge P, Gresty MA, Luxon LM (1998) Bilateral loss of vestibular function: clinical findings in 53 patients. *J Neurol* **245**: 314–21

Royal College of General Practitioners and Office of Population Census and Surveys (1986) *Morbidity Statistics from General Practice.* HMSO, London

Solomon D (2000) Distinguishing and treating causes of central vertigo. *Otolaryngol Clin North Am* **33**(3): 579–601

Strupp M, Brandt T (1999) Vestibular neuritis. *Adv Otorhinolaryngol* **55**: 111–36

Yardley L, Burgneay J, Andersson G, Owen N, Nazareth I (1998) Feasibility and effectiveness of providing vestibular rehabilitation for dizzy patients in the community. *Clin Otolaryngol* **23**: 442–8

# Chapter 16

# Cochlear and middle ear implants: advances for the hearing impaired

*CH Raine, J Martin*

We have entered into an era of surgical audiology with cochlear and middle ear implants. With both devices there are distinct phases of patient management – patient selection, surgery, programming and rehabilitation. These phases and issues relating to the implants themselves are considered in this chapter.

The surgical practice of cochlear implantation has developed considerably since its introduction into the UK in the late 1980s, whereas the middle ear implant is still in relative infancy. The cochlear implant stimulates the auditory nerve in patients with profound sensorineural deafness; the middle ear implant mechanically moves the ossicular chain in patients with moderate sensorineural loss. With such devices, patients now have an opportunity to hear when previously they failed to get benefit from conventional acoustic hearing aids.

## Cochlear implants

### History

The idea that electrical stimulation to the ear may be perceived as sound goes back some 200 years, although Djourno and Eyries provided the first detailed description of stimulating the auditory nerve in deafness in 1957. Initial implants, by today's standards, were simple single-channel systems, placed initially extracochlear, then eventually intracochlear. Single-channel devices were supplanted by multiple-channel devices in the early 1980s, based on enhanced spectral perception and enhanced recognition capabilities (Niparko and Wilson, 2000).

The cochlear implant is intended for people with sensorineural hearing loss who obtain limited benefit from appropriate binaural hearing aids (Summerfield and Marshall, 1995). Deafness occurs because of the failure of the cochlea to function. The hair cells are so damaged that they are incapable of transmitting meaningful signals to the auditory centre. The cochlear implant transforms soundwaves into electrical signals. The sound is picked up by a microphone usually worn at ear level and sent to the processor (*Figure 16.1*). This can be either worn on the body or behind the ear.

Various strategies of processing have been developed that produce both temporal and spatial coding. These codes are transmitted across the skin to the implanted receiver and electrodes (*Figure 16.1*).

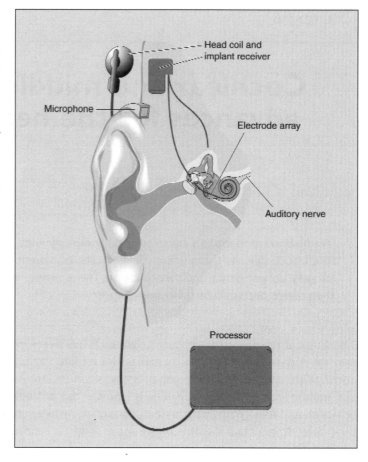

*Figure 16.1: Components of a cochlear implant.*

Surgery involves preparation of the bed for the receiver package, cortical mastoidectomy, posterior tympanotomy and finally entry into the cochlea usually by a separate cochleostomy into the scala tympani. The electrodes' signals stimulate the auditory nerve fibres within the modiolus to send information to the brain where they are interpreted as meaningful sound. Electrode and speech-processing designs have evolved to produce strategies that are associated with successively higher performance levels. In the UK, over 3500 patients have implants; worldwide, over 70000.

## Selection criteria

The selection of appropriate candidates for cochlear implants is critical to the success of these devices. Historically, the selection was vague, and the ill-defined criteria were:

⌘ bilateral sensorineural deafness
⌘ little or no benefit from hearing aids
⌘ no medical contraindications
⌘ well-motivated families with appropriate expectations.

With experience, further variables were identified that would affect performance. This led to the development of a multidisciplinary assessment. An organized listing of selection factors was developed by colleagues at the Manhattan Eye, Ear and Throat Hospital, known as the Children's Implant Profile (ChIP) (Hellman et al, 1991). This selection process has been adapted by a number of cochlear implant programmes, including the Yorkshire Cochlear Implant Service (YCIS).

Each factor on the ChIP (*Table 16.1*) is operationally defined and graded to the level of concern. The levels of concern vary from no concern, mild to moderate concern, and great concern.

The implant units in Bradford (YCIS) and Birmingham have devised a similar assessment profile for adults (*Table 16.2*).

Ten factors make up the profiles. The first four are static and are not amenable to direct remediation. The latter can be affected to a degree by intervention.

When dealing with prelingual or congenital deafness, age of intervention is important. Between 2–5 years of age would merit no concern because of the natural plasticity of the brain. The under-2-year olds are a moderate concern, as time is required to assess the degree of hearing loss, development and response to hearing aids. Certainly in recent years, the age at implantation has lowered. Children whose hearing loss is caused by meningitis should be referred promptly, regardless of age, to their nearest implant unit for 'fast tracking'.

Those over 8 years of age would be a great concern. Chute (1993) reported that adolescents were found to have minimal benefit from an implant 2 years after surgery. However, use of residual hearing, educational placement and the young person's own attitude towards hearing aids and cochlear implants are crucial factors for consideration.

Prelingually deafened adults have passed their period of maximum plasticity by the time they reach adulthood. Some may adapt to novel sensory input, but their progress is not ideal (National Institutes of Health Consensus Conference, 1995), and careful assessment is required (Manrique et al, 1995).

## Table 16.1: Children's implant profile

*Chronological age*

*Duration of deafness*

*Medical*

*Audiological*

Speech and language

Additional needs

Educational environment

Availability of support services

Family structure and support

Expectations: family and child

## Table 16.2: Adult implant profile

*Audiological*

*Functional hearing*

*Duration of deafness*

*Medical*

Additional needs

Communication skills

Support: home and work

Environment

Expectations: patient and family

Motivation and commitment

In postlingually deafened adults, the shorter the duration of profound deafness, the better the results with any assistive listening. With over 10 years of profound hearing loss, there is a marked decrease in cortical integrity, which in turn may be correlated to auditory nerve viability (Gantz et al, 1993). With increasing age, central presbyacusia compounds the hearing disability of many elderly patients and is a concern for cochlear implantation (Kelsall et al, 1995).

Good audiological information is required. Currently, cochlear implant teams are looking at aided thresholds of ≥50–55 dB at 2 and 4 kHz for paediatric candidacy, and at the results of Bamford–Kowal–Bench (BKB) open set sentence identification of >30% for adult candidacy.

Patients should be medically fit to undergo surgery. Radiological evaluation by computed tomography or magnetic resonance imaging scan will give information as to the likelihood of a full insertion of an electrode array. However, compressed and split electrodes systems have been developed to address the needs of congenitally abnormal or ossified cochlea (Bredberg et al, 1997).

Physical handicaps are not a specific contraindication. However, handicaps of a cognitive nature would be of great concern. Patients must be psychologically stable and be able to cope with all that is required with the process (Aplin, 1993). Patients with visual impairments may find that implantation promotes greater independence and improves quality of life (National Institutes of Health Consensus Conference, 1995).

With children, the educational setting and availability of support services are important. Local professionals must recognize the importance of the use of auditory–oral emphasis (Nevins and Chute, 1995). It is essential that this commitment is also obtained from the family. With appropriate counselling, the realistic benefits and limitations need to be appreciated. The process of habilitation takes a number of years. Children can achieve open set listening within 3–5 years. Adults who have been deaf for only a couple of years can achieve open set hearing within months or even weeks.

## Complications

Fortunately, complications of cochlear implantation are relatively uncommon (Gibbin et al, 2003). Postoperative infections are minimized with prophylactic antibiotics.

The facial nerve is at risk of damage when drilling the posterior tympanotomy. Facial nerve monitoring during surgery, especially when there are congenital anomalies, should be used (Raine et al, 1995).

The incidence of flap necrosis has reduced as implants have become smaller and incisions respect blood supply. The skin is under constant compression by the magnetic attraction between the implant and head coil. The strength of the magnet can be changed within the head coil to protect the skin.

The percentage cumulative survival data of implants, from the major implant companies, is in the high 90s. Re-implantation for failed devices does not usually present any significant difficulties. Non-use of an implant obviously has a major effect on healthcare economics (Summerfield and Marshall, 1995).

## Results

### Paediatric outcomes

With congenitally or perilingually deafened children, monitoring their auditory functional ability and speech intelligibility over time gives a good indication of outcome. The Category of Auditory Performance (Archbold et al, 1998) identifies eight levels of listening skill. Pre-implant, the majority of children are not aware of environmental sounds. After 3 years' implant use, they are able to understand everyday phrases without lip-reading. These are average scores, with many children being able to use the telephone within 3–4 years of receiving their implant (*Figure 16.2*).

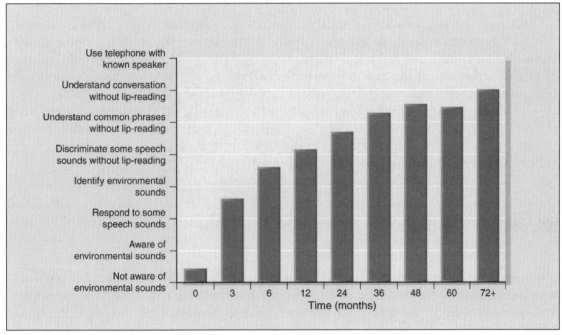

Figure 16.2: Category of auditory performance in children over time.

Because the development of intelligible speech is closely linked to hearing ability, children implanted at an early age have more potential to develop intelligible speech than those implanted at a later age.

### Adult outcomes

Quality-of-life questionnaires show that patients' confidence, relaxation and independence improve, whereas feelings of isolation and embarrassment decrease post-implant.

Postlingually deafened adults can show significant benefit. A study of over 800 patients (Blamey et al, 1996) showed that the duration of deafness had a strong negative effect on performance. Age at implantation had a slight negative effect on performance, increasing after

60 years of age. Age at onset of deafness had little effect up to the age of 60 years. The duration of implant use had a positive effect on performance, whereas aetiology had only a relatively weak effect on performance.

The YCIS outcomes report and detailed information about cochlea implants can be obtained from the British Cochlear Implant Group's website at www.bcig.org.

### The future

With the advent of universal neonatal screening for hearing impairment, children will be identified and assessed at an earlier age. Earlier intervention and oral communication are the most important known determinants of later speech perception (O'Donoghue et al, 2000).

Candidacy for implants are constantly under review. von Ilberg et al (1999) have shown that with appropriate surgical technique, residual hearing can be preserved. Patients with reasonable preservation of the low frequencies (≤65 dBHL at 125, 250 and 500 Hz) and with more classical losses at the higher frequencies (≥70 dBHL at 2 kHz and above) can benefit from a combination of electrical and auditory stimulation (EAS) (Kiefer et al, 2002).

Clinical studies are underway to evaluate benefit and quality-of-life issues around bilateral cochlear implants. They should also be considered in patients who have lost their hearing because of meningitis. Peri-modiolar electrodes are being designed and evaluated, as are various nerve growth factors to look at neural regeneration.

## Middle ear implants

There are a few different designs of middle ear implants (MEI). The principle of an implant is to enhance sound by mechanically moving the ossicles within the middle ear. The one implant that is mainly used in the UK is the Vibrant® Med-El Soundbridge® (Med-El, Innsbruck, Austria). This offers an alternative for patients with moderate to severe sensorineural hearing loss who experience limited benefit from conventional hearing aids. It is currently only used in adults.

The aims of such devices are to improve sound quality, both in quiet and noisy environments, and to reduce the problems of acoustic feedback (Lenarz et al, 1998). They are generally more comfortable to wear (Snik and Cremers, 1999). The occlusion effect of a standard hearing aid mould is eliminated. It also reduces the issue of maintenance as a result of cerumen and moisture accumulation.

The Vibrant® Soundbridge® is divided into external and internal parts, similar to a cochlear implant (*Figure 16.3*). The external part is called the audio processor. It contains the microphone, battery and electronics to convert sound into a signal suitable for transmission to the internal receiver.

The surgically implanted internal receiver connects to the floating mass transducer (FMT), which is clipped onto the incus in the middle ear (*Figure 16.4*).

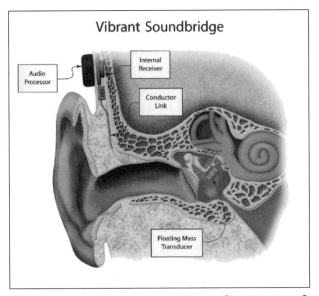

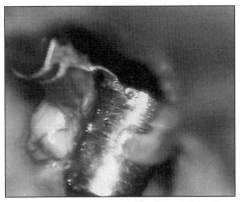

Figure 16.4: *Floating mass transducer on incus.*

Figure 16.3: *Components of the Vibrant® Soundbridge®. Reproduced with permission from Med-El (Med-El, Innsbruck, Austria).*

### Selection criteria

Patients should:

* be over 18 years of age
* have pure tone air conduction thresholds within the limits shown (*Figure 16.5*)
* have normal middle ear function
* have no previous middle ear disease or surgery
* have stable and symmetrical sensorineural hearing loss
* be dissatisfied with normal acoustic hearing aids
* be psychologically and emotionally stable.

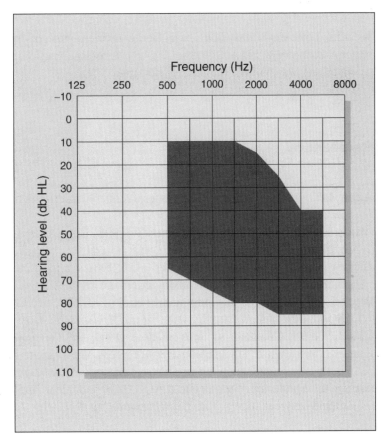

Figure 16.5. *Selection criteria for the Vibrant® Soundbridge®. dbHL = decibel hearing level.*

As with cochlear implants, the processor is not tuned in for a few weeks to allow the skin flap to settle. Complications of surgery are relatively similar to those of cochlear implants, except for the fact that the cochlea is not entered. Care must be taken when securing the FMT onto the incus.

## Results

Clinical trials are still underway, but initial reports have shown:

⌘ improved speech intelligibility
⌘ improved fidelity
⌘ no occlusion effect
⌘ no acoustic feedback.

Patients are also pleased with the aesthetics and the fact that wax or moist ears do not interfere with the working of the processor (vibrant@medel.com).

## The future

As with both implant systems, electronic refinements and improvements in microphone and battery technology will lead to the devices becoming totally implantable. New technologies are going a long way to help the hard of hearing.

# References

Aplin DY (1993) Psychological assessment of multi-channel cochlear implant patients. *J Laryngol Otol* **107**: 298–304

Archbold S, Lutman ME, Nikolopoulos T (1998) Categories of auditory performance: inter-user reliability. *Br J Audiol* **32**(1): 7–12

Blamey P, Arndt P, Bergeron F et al (1996) Factors affecting auditory performance of postlinguistically deaf adults using cochlear implants. *Audiol Neurootol* **1**(5): 293–306

Bredberg G, Lindstrom B, Lopponen H et al (1997) Electrodes for ossified cochleas. *Am J Otol* **18**(S6): 42–3

Chute P (1993) Cochlear implants in adolescents. *Adv Otorhinolaryngol* **48**: 210–15

Gantz B, Woodworth G, Knutson J et al (1993) Multivariate predictors of audiological success with multichannel cochlear implants. *Ann Otol Rhinol Laryngol* **102**: 909–16

Gibbin KP, Raine CH, Summerfield AQ (2003) Cochlear implantation — United Kingdom and Ireland surgical survey. *Cochlear Implants Int* **4**: 11–21

Hellman SA, Chute PM, Kretschner RE et al (1991) The development of a Children's Implant Profile. *Am Ann Deaf* **136**: 77–81

von Ilberg C, Keifer J, Tillein J et al (1999) Electric-acoustic stimulation of the auditory system. *Oto Rhino Laryngol* **61**: 334–40

Kelsall DC, Shallop JK, Burnelli T (1995) Cochlear implantation of the elderly. *Am J Otol* **15**: 573–87

Kiefer J, Tillien J, von Ilberg C et al (2002) Fundamental aspects and first results of the clinical application of combined electric and acoustic stimulation of the auditory system. In: Kubo T, Takahashi Y, Iwaki T, eds. *Cochlear Implants: an Update.* Kugler Publications, The Hague, The Netherlands: 569–76

Lenarz T, Weber BP, Mack KP et al (1998) The Vibrant Soundbridge system: a new kind of hearing aid for sensorineural hearing loss. 1: Function and initial clinical experiences. *Laryngorhinootologie* **77**: 247–55

Manrique N, Huarte A, Molina M et al (1995) Are cochlear implants indicated in prelingually deaf adults? *Ann Otol Rhinol Laryngol* **104**(S166): 192–4

Nevins ME, Chute PM (1995) Success of children with cochlear implants in mainstream educational settings. *Ann Otol Rhinol Laryngol* **104**(S166): 100–2

National Institutes of Health Consensus Conference (1995) Cochlear implants in adults and children. *JAMA* **274**: 1955–61

Niparko JK, Wilson BS (2000) History of cochlear implants. In: Niparko JK, Kirk KI, Mellon NK et al, eds. *Cochlear Implants: Principles and Practices.* Lippincott Williams and Wilkins, Philadelphia: 103–7

O'Donoghue G, Nikolopoulos TP, Archbold SM (2000) Determinants of speech perception in children after cochlear implantation. *Lancet* **356**: 466–8

Raine CH, Hussain SSM, Khan S et al (1995) Anomaly of the facial nerve and cochlear implantation. *Ann Otol Rhinol Laryngol* **104**(S166): 430–1

Snik AF, Cremers CW (1999) First audiometric results with the Vibrant Soundbridge, a semi-implantable hearing device for sensorineural hearing loss. *Audiology* **38**: 335–8

Summerfield AQ, Marshall DH (1995) *Cochlear Implants in the UK 1990–1994.* MRC Institute of Hearing Research, University of Nottingham. Her Majesty's Stationery Office, London

# Chapter 17

# Current trends in managing chronic middle ear disease

*John Hamilton*

Major advances in reconstruction continue to be made in the treatment of chronic middle ear disease, while little prophylaxis is available and indications for intervention remain in many cases controversial. This reflects our lack of knowledge of the true causes of such disease.

The most dramatic changes in patient care occur through new surgical procedures, particularly when new technologies are involved. Patients also benefit through refinements in selection for treatment and increases in surgical standards. Improved patient selection arises partly as a result of increased understanding of the natural history of disease and also from identifying treatment parameters that are most relevant to the patient. Surgical outcomes may also profit from changes in training and practice. In all these areas, recent progress has led to significant changes in middle ear surgery.

This chapter incorporates the most significant recent changes in the management of patients with chronic ear disease, and highlights areas where further progress remains desirable.

## Glue ear

The care of children with glue ear has been refined by an improved understanding of the natural history and social impact of the disease; the effectiveness of treatment has developed by focusing on outcome measures that are more relevant to patients as well as improving the scientific rigour of investigation.

While otitis media will affect most children (Teele et al, 1989), the majority of childhood middle ear effusions resolve spontaneously within 3 months (Fiellau-Nikolajsen, 1983). On the basis of this epidemiological information alone, it is clear that most episodes of glue ear do not require active intervention. Only those patients whose disease does not resolve should be considered for treatment. Currently the most reliable means for distinguishing this group is to identify those children whose disease does not improve in the medium term, generally considered to be approximately 3 months. This period of observation has been termed 'watchful waiting'.

This approach necessitates a delay before treatment, so other means of predicting persistence have been sought. Many risk factors have been associated with persistence (*Table 17.1*) (Daly, 1994). Only recently have the first group of these been proven to have true value for predicting persistence (Browning, 2001): season at attendance (high risk between July and December) and severity of hearing impairment (>30 dB hearing loss).

Paediatric glue ear is predominantly spontaneously remitting, so even placebo treatments can appear beneficial, and effective treatments can only be identified through prospective controlled and blinded research.

Based on audiological outcomes, such work has shown that medical treatments can provide only short-term (weeks) improvement in hearing (Williams et al, 1993). Insertion of tympanic membrane ventilation tubes can provide a medium-term (months) benefit (Effective Health Care, 1992), and adenoidectomy provides a longer-term benefit (Effective Health Care, 1992). Less invasive treatment with hearing aids remains unproven but appears to provide long-term symptomatic benefit (Flanagan et al, 1996), especially for children with ultra-persistent glue ear, many of whom have underlying problems such as cleft palate or Down's syndrome.

Not all children with impaired audiological outcomes have difficulties, and research using outcomes more closely related to disability has been performed. Bennett et al (2001) have shown that behavioural problems and developmental delay can be detected into the teens in children who had persistent glue ear in earlier childhood.

Attempts have been made to determine how these effective treatments can be most appropriately used (Agency for Health Care Policy and Research, 1994; Bluestone and Klein, 1994). The individual child's circumstances prevent the formulation of an acceptable systematic programme of treatment. When to act, when not to act and how best to act are questions that are influenced by the child's surroundings, support and personality. Optimum treatment can only be offered after listening to the child and carers; it is therefore vital in the management of glue ear that time in clinic is provided to do this.

## Table 17.1: Risk factors for glue ear

Craniofacial abnormality

Down's syndrome

Cleft palate

Cilial abnormality

Large adenoids

Family history

Male sex

Season

Bottle feeding

Day care

Upper respiratory tract infection

Inhalant allergy

Socioeconomic status

Parental smoking

Damp housing

Modified from Haggard and Hughes (1991)

# Perforated ears

Techniques for surgical closure of the perforated tympanic membrane were established just over 40 years ago. Improvements in the short-term results of tympanoplasty have followed from techniques to improve access to the tympanic membrane and from improved patient selection. There is no clear understanding of the long-term results of tympanic membrane surgery.

Audit reveals that the results of repair for anterior perforations are often worse than for posterior perforations (Halik and Smyth, 1988). The reason for poor results in anterior tympanic membrane surgery is that there is often poor access to this area. When viewed through the external meatus, the anterior part of the annulus can be hidden by the anterior wall of the ear canal, as the canal is six times as long as it is wide and also curves anteriorly and inferiorly (Williams and Warwick, 1980). Exposure of the entire tympanic membrane by widening the canal surgically has resulted in uniformly excellent results of tympanoplasty regardless of the site or size of perforation.

There is no evidence regarding which material provides the most effective closure. Temporalis fascia and tragal perichondrium are widely used in the UK, while in Germany thinned cartilage is popular (Zahnert et al, 2000). Cartilage has also been reported to provide good long-term results in repair of children's perforated ears (El-Hennawi, 2001). Most studies indicate that the repair of tympanic membrane perforations in children results in a higher rate of failure in the medium to long term than in adults (Lancaster et al, 1999).

There exists only one paper with robust statistics on the long-term results of tympanic membrane repair (Halik and Smyth, 1988). Life table analysis showed that the percentage of normal tympanic membranes fell from 94% at 1 year to 74% at 10 years. This study included procedures on children under 10 years of age as well as patients with cholesteatoma, so it is likely that it underestimates the benefit of surgery. Nonetheless, the paper raises some as yet unanswered questions about the evaluation of surgical intervention as well as the processes underlying the spontaneous deterioration of the repaired ear.

# Retraction pockets

Inflammation of the tympanic membrane sometimes results in loss of the fibrous layer. Absence of this strong layer can cause the affected area to collapse or retract. Treatment of such retraction pockets has caused great controversy, as their behaviour has been unpredictable. Many cause no symptoms and can even heal back to normal. Some eventually perforate, some cause erosion of the ossicles, thereby reducing hearing, and some can progress to become cholesteatoma. Sade (2001) has quantified these events and has demonstrated that only 1% of retraction pockets will progress to become cholesteatoma.

The treatment of retraction pockets remains highly controversial. Maw and Bawden (1994) have shown that grommet insertion does not act as a prophylaxis against the development of retractions. Most surgeons will operate if there is evidence of advancing disease, such as ongoing symptoms, overt inflammation or progressive ossicular erosion. Sade (2001) has also demonstrated that the retraction pockets most likely to advance are those associated with a small mastoid.

The surgical treatment of many retraction pockets has been greatly simplified (Ars, 1991). Ars has shown that simply excising the pocket will result in subsequent spontaneous closure of the defect, provided that an air pressure difference across the tympanic membrane is prevented with the use of a mini-grommet. Sharp and Robinson (1992) confirmed that this simple technique gives good results. In a small percentage of cases, the retraction pocket returns. It can then be treated by conventional reinforcement myringoplasty.

## Cholesteatoma

Successful treatment of cholesteatoma requires the entire removal of the disease, prevention of its return, reconstruction of an ear robust enough to withstand exposure to water and the preservation or reconstruction of hearing. The earliest procedures aimed only at effecting the first two of these; the means of achieving a robust ear continues to excite great controversy today, while the reconstruction of a greatly damaged ossicular chain remains a challenge.

Cholesteatoma can insinuate itself into all the interstices of the complex temporal bone anatomy. It can grow behind structures the surgeon does not wish to displace, and can be firmly adherent to the delicate ossicular chain. For these reasons, and also because even microscopic fragments can re-grow, it has been difficult to completely eradicate cholesteatoma with conventional instruments (Robinson, 1997).

The development of visible light lasers, which can be transmitted down optical fibres, has marked a significant advance in the reduction of such residual disease as it can eradicate disease in all the above circumstances (Hamilton, 2001). The laser can vaporize cholesteatoma in spaces difficult to reach conventionally. It also can vaporize cholesteatoma adherent to the ossicles, including the stapes, without imparting any damaging movement to the inner ear. Moreover, it can be used to heat and denature all the surfaces with which the cholesteatoma has had contact, thereby eliminating retained microscopic fragments. Using a potassium-titanyl-phosphate (KTP) laser as part of a two-stage intact canal wall technique over a 30-month period, there were no cases of residual disease at the second look operation (Hamilton, 2001).

Various techniques have been developed to increase the stability of the ear after cholesteatoma surgery. These culminated in the preservation of the ear canal, as pioneered by Jansen in 1958, and to this day surgeons argue about the merits and disadvantages of 'canal wall up' or 'canal wall down' surgery.

The vanguard of cholesteatoma surgeons in the 1970s noted that the intact canal wall technique at that time resulted in a high incidence of both residual and recurrent disease (Cody and Taylor, 1977). Techniques to reconstruct canal wall defects (Perkins, 1976) and the introduction of an essential second look operation to check for residual disease (Wright, 1977) brought continued life to canal wall up surgery.

A staged technique using bone pate to reconstruct the annulus has been studied in a cohort followed up for over 10 years. Life table analysis of this group has shown a recurrence rate at 10 years of less than 3% (J Hamilton, unpublished data, 2000).

# Ossicular surgery

Improving ossicular surgery is one of the great remaining challenges for otology. Sound transmission after surgical reconstruction of the ossicular chain remains variable and generally suboptimal. Altering the surgical outcome measure has, however, improved the ability to predict the benefit to the patient of ossiculoplasty. Outcome measures were previously rather conceptual and principally of technical interest; now they are increasingly expressed in terms of patient benefit and more useful in determining the value of surgery.

In the past, the difference between the ipsilateral air conduction and bone conduction thresholds, the air–bone gap, was used to gauge the success of surgery. It was useful as a measure of the technical success in restoring the middle ear hearing apparatus but masked any associated inner ear damage and was of little value in measuring patient benefit. The ipsilateral postoperative air conduction threshold alone has proven more relevant to the latter. Consideration of the effect of the contralateral hearing has also provided great insight into the value of ossicular surgery.

Combining these parameters gave rise to the Belfast rules of thumb (*Table 17.2*) (Smyth and Patterson, 1985). The Belfast rules of thumb were the first means of evaluating the effect of surgery on binaural hearing ability. This permitted a much more reliable guide to the extent to which patients' hearing could be relieved by surgery. Alternative benefit measures have been developed (Browning et al, 1991), and the insight provided by these techniques is useful in planning ossicular surgery.

For instance, this analysis has demonstrated that the extent of damage to the ossicular chain is an important determinant of adequate hearing reconstruction after cholesteatoma surgery. An intact chain, or a chain reconstructed after loss of only the lenticular process of the incus, leads to satisfying hearing in 80% of cases. By contrast, reconstruction after loss of the stapes superstructure results in satisfying hearing in only 40% (Hamilton and Robinson, 2000).

The importance of any associated sensorineural hearing loss in an operated ear when the opposite ear is normal should not be underestimated, as it may nullify the benefits of even the most technically excellent ossiculoplasty (Hamilton and Robinson, 2000).

Ossicular surgery has been an early area in which changes in patterns of practice have been advocated. For instance, stapedotomy, the surgical procedure for improving hearing in otosclerosis, provides a reliable improvement in hearing in the hands of experts. It is, however, a demanding operation that can have significant associated morbidity. As clinical governance takes effect and regulations are applied in keeping with the Kennedy report (The Stationery Office, 2001), it is likely that stapes surgery will be concentrated in the hands of fewer individuals, and only surgeons regularly performing the procedure will treat patients. To some extent, this has already happened.

| Table 17.2: The Belfast rules of thumb |
| --- |
| ⌘ To ensure that the patient will benefit from surgery to improve hearing, the operated ear must reach an air conduction level of 30 dB hearing loss for the speech frequencies |
| ⌘ The operated ear must reach an air conduction level within 15 dB of the other ear |

The increased association of applied mathematicians and materials scientists with research otologists is starting to result in new approaches to designing ossicular prostheses, estimating their behaviour and planning their disposition.

Materials for use in the ossicular chain are chosen according to the response, if any, that they invoke from the middle ear, as well as their dynamic mechanical properties. Titanium, for instance, has a density similar to bone (Huettenbrink, 2000), and the stiffness of a titanium prosthesis can be adjusted according to its shape. Earlier observations have shown bone to conform well to the shape of adjacent titanium, ensuring a secure fit between the two surfaces.

The optimum shape and location of prostheses is likely to be determined by finite element analysis and laser Doppler vibrometry. Finite element analysis (Funnell and Laszlo, 1978) is a means of modelling complex mechanical systems as networks of interconnected discrete elements. Among many applications in middle ear mechanics, it has been used to predict the mechanism of action of an ossicular prosthesis (Williams and Lesser, 1992) and to estimate the optimum positioning of another prosthesis (Asai et al, 1999). Laser Doppler vibrometry can measure the vibration of objects whose movement has an amplitude less than the wavelength of light (Michelsen and Larsen, 1978).

Commercial instruments to exploit this technique have flourished because of their value to the automobile industry. Recently they have been applied to the middle ear, and laser Doppler vibrometry has revealed the exquisite manner in which the ossicular chain moves under the effect of incident sound (Decraemer and Khanna, 2000). This technique has also been used to test the vibration of ossicular prostheses (Lord et al, 2000). The use of finite element analysis to predict behaviour and laser Doppler vibrometry to confirm it provides the basis for optimizing ossicular surgery in the future (Eibner et al, 1999).

## Hearing aids

As with other areas involving computers, advances in hearing aid technology are rapid at present. Digital and 'completely in the ear' aids are widely available from private dispensers. The National Institute for Clinical Excellence judged that there was insufficient evidence to justify NHS provision for digital aids (NICE, 2000). As a consequence, a government-sponsored trial of the performance of digital against analogue aids was undertaken. The results favoured digital hearing aids, and these are now dispensed by the NHS.

Some patients with congenital disorders of the external or middle ears are not able to wear conventional hearing aids. Surgery or conventional aids similarly cannot help patients with complex acquired external or middle ear disorders. In the past, such patients could only be offered hearing aids that stimulated the hearing by pressing firmly against the skull through the scalp – these were both unsightly and uncomfortable. Osseo-integration allows stimulation of hearing through a titanium platform anchored to the skull so that there is no pressure on the scalp (Tjellstrom et al, 1981). As patients are not continually reminded of their presence, they find such bone-anchored hearing aids acceptable (Mylanus et al, 1995).

Implantable hearing aids for sensorineural hearing loss have also been developed (Snik et al, 2001). Much of the funding for the investigation of ossicular motion by laser Doppler vibrometry has been provided by organizations interested in developing implantable hearing aids. This is because the implanted aid has an element that is attached to the ossicular chain, and the means of attachment and its location critically affect the performance of such devices. Until reliable long-term results are available, these aids should be considered experimental.

## The future

It is always entertaining to speculate on the nature of surgery in the future. Consideration of the underlying causes of change allows more latitude into such speculation. Thus, the management of patients with chronic middle ear disease is likely to progress under the following influences.

Research to reduce the gaps in our understanding of the physiology of the middle ear as well as the underlying causes of chronic middle ear disease will allow the indications for intervention in middle ear disease to become more focused. Research into the means for effecting such changes will doubtless progress.

It is equally likely that there will continue to be important changes regarding who it is considered appropriate to treat and who will perform the surgery. These may result from a more formal assessment of surgeons' performance and changes in public involvement with treatment.

New technologies and procedures, hard proof of efficacy, rigorous audit and changes in working patterns are all expensive. Although other factors may modify progress, availability of funding is likely to control the future rate of change of the management of chronic middle ear disease.

## References

Agency for Health Care Policy and Research (1994) *Otitis Media with Effusion in Young Children.* Clinical Practice Guideline 12. US Public Health Service, Washington

Ars BMJ (1991) Tympanic membrane-retraction pockets. In: Charachon R, Garcia-Ibanez E, eds. *Long-term Results and Indications in Otology and Otoneurosurgery.* Kugler Publications, Amsterdam: 19–31

Asai M, Huber AM, Goode RL (1999) Analysis of the best site on the stapes footplate for ossicular reconstruction. *Acta Otolaryngol* **119**: 356–61

Bennett KE, Haggard MP, Silva PA, Stewart IA (2001) Behaviour and developmental effects of otitis media with effusion into the teens. *Arch Dis Child* **85**: 91–5

Bluestone CD, Klein JO (1994) Clinical practice guideline on otitis media with effusion in young children: strengths and weaknesses. *Otolaryngol Head Neck Surg* **112**: 507–11

Browning GG, Gatehouse S, Swan IR (1991) The Glasgow Benefit Plot: a new method for reporting benefits from middle ear surgery. *Laryngoscope* **101**: 180–5

Browning GG (2001) Watchful waiting in childhood otitis media with effusion. *Clin Otolaryngol* **26**: 263–4

Cody DT, Taylor WF (1977) Mastoidectomy for acquired cholesteatoma: long-term results. In: McCabe BF, Sade J, Abramson M, eds. *Cholesteatoma. First International Conference.* Aesculapius Publishing Company, Birmingham, Al: 337–51

Daly K (1994) Risk factors for otitis media sequelae and chronicity. *Ann Otol Rhinol Laryngol* **103**: 39–42

Decraemer WF, Khanna SM (2000) Three dimensional vibration of the ossicular chain in the cat. Vibration measurements by laser techniques: advances and applications. *SPIE* **4072**: 401–11

Effective Health Care (1992) The treatment of persistent glue ear in children. *Effective Health Care Bull* **4**: 1–16

Eibner A, Freitag HG, Burkhardt C et al (1999) Dynamics of middle ear prostheses — simulations and measurements. *Audiol Neuro Otol* **4**: 178–84

El-Hennawi DM (2001) Cartilage-perichondrium composite graft in pediatric tympanoplasty. *Int J Pediatr Otorhinolaryngol* **59**: 1–5

Fiellau-Nikolajsen M (1983) Typanometry and secretory otitis media. *Acta Otolaryngologica (Stockh) Suppl*: 394

Flanagan PM, Knight LC, Thomas A, Browning S, Aymat A, Clayton MI (1996) Hearing aids and glue ear. *Clin Otolaryngol* **21**: 297–300

Funnell WRJ, Laszlo CA (1978) Modelling of the cat eardrum as a thin shell using the finite element method. *J Acoust Soc Am* **63**: 1461–7

Haggard MP, Hughes E (1991) *Screening Children's Hearing.* HMSO, London: 41–66

Halik JJ, Smyth GDL (1988) Long-term results of tympanic membrane repair. *Otolaryngol Head Neck Surg* **98**: 162–9

Hamilton JW (2001) The KTP laser in cholesteatoma surgery. In: Oswal V, Jovanovic S, Remacle M, eds. *Lasers in Otorhinolaryngology.* Kugler Publications, Amsterdam

Hamilton JW, Robinson JM (2000) Short-term and long-term hearing results after middle ear surgery. In: Rosowski JJ, Merchant SN, eds. *The Function and Mechanics of Normal, Diseased and Reconstructed Middle Ears.* Kugler Publications, The Hague, The Netherlands

Huettenbrink K-B (2000) Zur Rekonstruktion des Schallleitungsapparates unter biomechanischen Gesichtspunkten. *Laryngo Rhino Otol* **79**: S23–S51

Lancaster JL, Makura ZG, Porter G, McCormick M (1999) Paediatric tympanoplasty. *J Laryngol Otol* **113**: 628–32

Lord RM, Mills RP, Abel EW (2000) An anatomically shaped incus prosthesis for reconstruction of the ossicular chain. *Hear Res* **145**: 141–8

Maw AR, Bawden R (1994) Tympanic membrane atrophy, scarring, atelectasis and attic retraction in persistent, untreated otitis media with effusion and following ventilation tube insertion. *Int J Pediatr Otorhinolaryngol* **30**: 189–204

Michelsen A, Larsen ON (1978) Biophysics of the Eusiferan ear. *J Comp Physiol* **123**: 193–203

Mylanus EAM, Snik AF, Cremers CW (1995) The bone anchored *vs* the conventional hearing aid, the patients' opinion. *Arch Otolaryngol Head Neck Surg* **121**: 421–5

National Institute for Clinical Excellence (2000) *Guidance on Hearing Aid Technology.* NICE Technology Appraisal Guidance No. 8. National Institute for Clinical Excellence, London

Perkins R (1976) Tympanomastoid reconstruction: an operative procedure for anatomical and functional restoration of the radicalized ear. *Laryngoscope* **86**: 416–30

Robinson JM (1997) Cholesteatoma: skin in the wrong place. *J R Soc Med* **90**: 93–5

Sade J (2001) Hyperectasis: the hyperinflated tympanic membrane: the middle ear as an actively controlled system. *Otol Neurotol* **22**: 133–9

Sharp JF, Robinson JM (1992) Treatment of tympanic membrane retraction pockets by excision. A prospective study. *J Laryngol Otol* **106**: 771–2

Snik AF, Mylanus EA, Cremers CW et al (2001) Multicenter audiometric results with the Vibrant Soundbridge, a semi-implantable hearing device for sensorineural hearing impairment. *Otolaryngol Clin North Am* **34**: 373–88

Smyth GD, Patterson CC (1985) Results of middle ear reconstruction: do patients and surgeons agree? *Am J Otol* **6**: 276–9

Teele DW, Klein JO, Rosner B and the Greater Boston Otitis Media Study Group (1989) Epidemiology of otitis media during the first 7 years of life in children in Greater Boston: a prospective cohort study. *J Infect Dis* **160**: 83–94

The Stationery Office (2001) Public inquiry into children's heart surgery at the Bristol Royal Infirmary 1984-1995. In: *Learning from Bristol*. Cmnd 5207. The Stationery Office, London

Tjellstrom A, Lindstrom J, Hallen O, Albrektsson T, Branemark P-I (1981) Osseointegrated titanium implants in the temporal bone. A clinical study on bone anchored hearing aids. *Am J Otol* **2**: 304–10

Williams PL, Warwick R (1980) *Gray's Anatomy*. 36th edn. Churchill Livingstone, Edinburgh

Williams KR, Lesser TH (1992) A dynamic and natural frequency analysis of the Fisch II spandrel using the finite element method. *Clin Otolaryngol* **17**: 261–70

Williams RL, Chalmers TC, Stange KC, Chalmers FT, Bowlin SJ (1993) The use of antibiotics in preventing recurrent acute otitis media and in treating otitis media with effusion. A meta-analytic attempt to resolve the brouhaha. *JAMA* **270**: 1344–51

Wright WK (1977) A concept for the management of otitic cholesteatomas. In: McCabe BF, Sade J, Abramson M, eds. *Cholesteatoma*. First International Conference. Aesculapius Publishing Company, Birmingham, AL: 374–8

Zahnert T, Huettenbrink K-B, Murbe D, Bornitz M (2000) Experimental investigations of the use of cartilage in tympanic membrane reconstruction. *Am J Otol* **21**: 322–8

# Index